PreTest®

Behavioral Sciences

Notice

Medicine is an ever-changing science. As new research and clinical experience broaden our knowledge, changes in treatment and drug therapy are required. The editor and the publisher of this work have checked with sources believed to be reliable in their efforts to provide information that is complete and generally in accord with the standards accepted at the time of publication. However, in view of the possibility of human error or changes in medical sciences, neither the editors nor the publisher nor any other party who has been involved in the preparation or publication of this work warrants that the information contained herein is in every respect accurate or complete, and they are not responsible for any errors or omissions or for the results obtained from use of such information. Readers are encouraged to confirm the information contained herein with other sources. For example and in particular, readers are advised to check the product information sheet included in the package of each drug they plan to administer to be certain that the information contained in this book is accurate and that changes have not been made in the recommended dose or in the contraindications for administration. This recommendation is of particular importance in connection with new or infrequently used drugs.

Behavioral Sciences

PreTest®
Self-Assessment
and Review

Seventh Edition

Editor

Evan G. Pattishall, Jr., Ph.D., M.D.

*Dean Emeritus and Professor Emeritus of Behavioral Science,
Health and Human Development
College of Health and Human Development
The Pennsylvania State University
University Park, Pennsylvania*

 McGraw-Hill
Health Professions Division
PreTest® Series

New York   St. Louis   San Francisco   Auckland
Bogotá   Caracas   Lisbon   London   Madrid
Mexico City   Milan   Montreal   New Delhi
San Juan   Singapore   Sydney   Tokyo   Toronto

McGraw-Hill

A Division of The McGraw·Hill Companies

Behavioral Sciences: PreTest® Self-Assessment and Review, 7/e
Copyright © 1996 by McGraw-Hill, Inc. All rights reserved. Printed in the United States of America. Except as permitted under the Copyright Act of 1976, no part of this publication may be reproduced or distributed in any form or by any means, or stored in a data base or retrieval system, without the prior written permission of the publisher.

1 2 3 4 5 6 7 8 9 0   DOCDOC   9 9 8 7 6 5

ISBN 0-07-052084-4

The editors were Gail Gavert and Bruce MacGregor.
The production supervisor was Gyl A. Favours.
R.R. Donnelley & Sons was printer and binder.
This book was set in Times Roman by Digitype.

Library of Congress Cataloging-in-Publication Data
Behavioral sciences : PreTest self-assessment and review / edited by Evan
  G. Pattishall, Jr. — 7th ed.
    p.   cm.
  Includes bibliographical references.
  ISBN 0-07-052084-4 (pbk.)
  1. Psychology—Examinations, questions, etc.   2. Social sciences—
Examinations, questions, etc.   I. Pattishall, Evan G. (Evan Gradick), 1921–
BF78.B43   1996
150'.76—dc20   95–5754

Contents

Contents

Introduction

Each *PreTest® Self-Assessment and Review* allows medical students to comprehensively and conveniently assess and review their knowledge of a particular basic science, in this instance Behavioral Sciences. The 500 questions parallel the format and degree of difficulty of the questions found in the United States Medical Licensing Examination (USMLE) Step 1. Practicing physicians who want to hone their skills before USMLE Step 3 or recertification may find this to be a good beginning in their review process.

Each question is accompanied by an answer, a paragraph explanation, and a specific page reference to an appropriate textbook or journal article. A bibliography listing sources can be found following the last chapter of this text.

An effective way to use this PreTest® is to allow yourself one minute to answer each question in a given chapter. As you proceed, indicate your answer beside each question. By following this suggestion, you approximate the time limits imposed by the Step.

After you finish going through the questions in the section, spend as much time as you need verifying your answers and carefully reading the explanations provided. Pay special attention to the explanations for the questions you answered incorrectly—but read every explanation. The editor of this material has designed the explanations to reinforce and supplement the information tested by the questions. If you feel you need further information about the material covered, consult and study the references indicated.

PreTest®

Behavioral Sciences

Biologic Correlates of Behavior

DIRECTIONS: Each question below contains five suggested responses. Select the **one best** response to each question.

1. In studying the interaction of psychological stress and DNA repair, suppressed DNA repair was found in persons with

(A) chronic stress more often than those with acute stress
(B) low distress over an extended period of time
(C) a diagnosis of major depression
(D) increased anxiety and depression from bereavement
(E) recently diagnosed cancer

2. Clinical features of major depressive disorders suggest a defect in the

(A) frontal lobes
(B) pituitary
(C) hippocampus
(D) hypothalamus
(E) corpus callosum

3. The pituitary secretion of endorphins is closely linked to the secretion of adrenocorticotropic hormone (ACTH) so that endorphins facilitate the ability to respond to

(A) retarded growth
(B) severe hypertension
(C) stress
(D) chronic pain
(E) tachycardia

4. Dream deprivation in humans tends to produce

(A) impaired performance on simple verbal tasks with no emotional content
(B) less total need for dream sleep
(C) major impairment of psychological functions
(D) retardation of formation of memory
(E) integration of emotional material with memories of other experiences

5. A 47-year-old, recently divorced, male bookkeeper experienced a gnawing epigastric pain over the past week, very similar to a bout of pain he had experienced a year ago and which was diagnosed as a duodenal ulcer. The factor most likely responsible for the exacerbation of his ulcer is

(A) expression of a characteristic personality
(B) chronic anxiety and stress
(C) snacking on food
(D) socioeconomic status
(E) occupation

6. In the treatment of psychophysiologic disorders, minor tranquilizers can be expected to

(A) result in long-term improvement
(B) reduce interpersonal dilemmas
(C) produce a mild stimulus
(D) be used without development of tolerance
(E) reduce high levels of stress

7. The diathesis-stress model of psychophysiologic disorders postulates the presence of which of the following major factors?

(A) Inadequate coping style
(B) Individual response stereotype
(C) Lack of health belief resolution
(D) Adequate homeostatic restraints
(E) Unconditioned stimulus

8. Harry Harlow's work with inanimate surrogate mothers for monkeys suggests that the early experience critical to the ultimate development of "love" is

(A) positive reinforcement
(B) protection from danger
(C) contact comfort
(D) need-reduction by nursing
(E) sexual stimulation

9. The hormone with the greatest role in aggression is

(A) thyroxine
(B) testosterone
(C) estrogen
(D) progesterone
(E) aldosterone

10. When an inactive substance or condition induces a therapeutic change, the procedure (result) is called

(A) modulated conditioning
(B) reaction formation
(C) placebo effect
(D) fantasy reaction
(E) nonpharmaceutical reaction

11. The most common organic explanation for a sleep disturbance in a healthy person is

(A) disruption of normal circadian rhythms
(B) accumulation of hepatic enzymes
(C) the inevitable consequences of high activity
(D) suppressed REM sleep
(E) misuse of hypnotics

12. The relationship between social and biologic processes in the generation of behavior has historically been classified by which of the following terms?

(A) Classically conditioned
(B) Organic and functional
(C) Genetic and familial
(D) Neuropathologic and sociopathologic
(E) Psychoanalytic and dynamic

13. The use of relaxation techniques for stress reduction affects diabetic patients by producing

(A) increased levels of plasma cortisol
(B) increased sensitivity to insulin
(C) increased glucose-stimulated secretion of insulin
(D) significant improvement in glucose tolerance
(E) no significant change in requirements for exogenous insulin

14. Dream deprivation is most apt to produce

(A) a rebound phenomenon of increased dreaming
(B) an increase in anxiety and irritability
(C) acceleration of memory formation of emotionally toned words
(D) a decrement in intellectual function
(E) a temporary increase in nightmares

15. Which of the following statements about natural killer cells is true?

(A) Their activity increases with the secretion of corticosteroids through the hypothalamic-pituitary-adrenal axis
(B) They play a role in inhibition of tumor growth
(C) They are ineffective in deterring the spread of distant cancer
(D) Their activity increases under conditions of psychosocial stress
(E) None of the above

16. Coping effort associated with negative emotions, such as embarrassment or feeling harassed, results in preferential secretion of

(A) corticotropin
(B) norepinephrine
(C) epinephrine
(D) catecholamines
(E) cortisol

DIRECTIONS: Each numbered question or incomplete statement below is NEGATIVELY phrased. Select the **one best** lettered response.

17. All the following endocrine glands are subject to control by the brain EXCEPT the

(A) pancreatic islets
(B) pituitary
(C) parathyroid
(D) thyroid
(E) adrenal

18. Of the following hormones, the LEAST important in influencing sexual behavior is

(A) luteinizing hormone releasing factor
(B) oxytocin
(C) estradiol
(D) testosterone
(E) androstenedione

19. All the following are common forms of psychophysiologic disorders EXCEPT

(A) bronchial asthma
(B) dysmenorrhea
(C) headache
(D) diabetes
(E) neurodermatitis

20. When an axon is cut, all the following events take place EXCEPT

(A) there is a rapid local degeneration of the axon and myelin sheath
(B) macrophages from the general circulation are unable to enter the area to phagocytose axonal debris
(C) proliferation of fibrous astrocytes forms a glial scar around the zone of trauma
(D) scarring can block the course taken by the regenerating axons
(E) degeneration spreads in both directions along the axon from the zone of trauma

21. Immunocompetence can be suppressed by all the following EXCEPT

(A) the endocrine system
(B) chronic stress of long duration
(C) the central nervous system
(D) the autonomic nervous system
(E) psychosocial factors

22. All the following statements on the influence of environment on brain structure and behavior are true EXCEPT

(A) the structure of the brain is to an important degree specified by genetic and developmental processes

(B) the pattern of interconnections between neurons is influenced considerably by experience

(C) there is very little evidence for the notion of the critical period in the development of normal social and perceptual competence

(D) at certain stages in its development, the integrative action of the brain and its cellular structure are dependent upon the brain's interaction with its environment

(E) the action of the environment on the brain varies with age

23. Antibody titers to latent viruses, e.g., Epstein-Barr or herpes simplex, can be increased at least initially by all the following EXCEPT

(A) relaxation training

(B) immunosuppressive chemotherapy

(C) the stress of academic examinations

(D) loneliness

(E) sustained noise

24. Psychosocial stress increases the secretion of catecholamines and thus induces an increase in a number of cardiovascular pathogenic phenomena. All the following are increased EXCEPT

(A) damage to intima of coronary arteries

(B) blood pressure and heart rate

(C) blood lipids

(D) first-degree AV block

(E) ventricular arrhythmias

25. Hyperventilation from anxiety, threat, or fear results in all the following EXCEPT

(A) reduced CO_2 in the blood

(B) reduced acid level in the blood

(C) increased sympathetic activity

(D) increased risk of cardiac arrhythmia

(E) increased oxygen supplied to brain tissue

26. Studies of the effects of acute and chronic stress in humans indicate that the activity of all the following components of the immune system are decreased EXCEPT

(A) polymorphonuclear granulocytes

(B) lymphocyte T-cell cytotoxicity

(C) production of interferon

(D) latent virus antibody titers

(E) activity of natural killer cells

27. Over time, vigorous exercise results in all the following EXCEPT

(A) increased high-density lipoprotein cholesterol (HDL-C)
(B) decreased low-density lipoprotein cholesterol (LDL-C)
(C) decreased very low-density lipoprotein cholesterol (VLDL-C)
(D) decreased total cholesterol
(E) increased triglycerides

28. The left hemisphere of the brain is generally associated with each of the following functions EXCEPT

(A) language acquisition
(B) affective aspects of language
(C) mathematical reasoning
(D) finger dexterity
(E) vocalization

29. Dynorphin, a natural brain endorphin, has all the following characteristics EXCEPT that it is

(A) 50 times more potent than any other known endorphin
(B) 200 times more potent than morphine
(C) able to bind to pain receptors with great specificity
(D) a producer of tolerance and dependence
(E) clinically useful in more severe pain problems

30. Of the following laboratory studies, all have found evidence of brain dysfunction in 50 percent or more of persons with schizophrenia EXCEPT

(A) lactate infusion test
(B) neurologic examination for soft signs (e.g., grasp and rooting reflexes)
(C) abnormal eye pursuit test
(D) impairment in neuropsychological tests
(E) abnormal electroencephalogram (EEG)

31. Consumption of alcohol is associated with all the following EXCEPT

(A) inhibition of mobility of macrophages
(B) inhibition of proliferation of T cells
(C) inhibition of cytotoxicity of T cells
(D) inhibition of production of antibodies
(E) damage to the thymus

32. Research on rapid eye movement (REM) sleep patterns shows all the following findings EXCEPT that

(A) a newborn baby spends more than 50 percent of sleep time in REM sleep

(B) under normal circumstances, 80 percent of the adult sleep cycle consists of REM sleep

(C) deep sleep begins to be replaced with longer periods of REM sleep after the age of 30

(D) the amount of REM sleep determines the amount of actual rest

(E) when REM sleep is interrupted consistently, tiredness and neurotic tendencies develop

33. A lesion of the axons of motor neurons that innervate skeletal muscle (lower motor neurons) will result in all the following consequences EXCEPT

(A) paralysis of individual muscles on the side of the lesion

(B) a paradoxical increase in reflex activity

(C) reduction in muscle mass (atrophy)

(D) decrease in muscle tone

(E) sealing off of the axoplasm

34. When one faces stressors for which there is no apparent coping strategy, one manifests vigilant inaction, which results in all the following EXCEPT

(A) decreased skeletal movement

(B) increased blood pressure

(C) vagus nerve–mediated bradycardia

(D) increased levels of corticotropin (ACTH) and cortisol

(E) increased levels of brain norepinephrine

35. All the following medications affect sexual function by decreasing arousal EXCEPT

(A) tricyclics

(B) amphetamines

(C) phenothiazines

(D) alpha-methyldopa

(E) guanethidine

36. All the following statements about sleeping pills are correct EXCEPT

(A) they lose their effectiveness in about 2 weeks

(B) barbiturates gradually lead to an increase in hepatic enzymes

(C) patients develop tolerance for benzodiazepines much less rapidly than for pentobarbital

(D) barbiturates enhance REM sleep

(E) there is often a broad cross-tolerance to other hypnotics

37. All the following response patterns will usually accompany dreaming EXCEPT

(A) electroencephalographic desynchrony
(B) more visual imagery during non-REM sleep
(C) rapid eye movements
(D) loss of sternocleidomastoid tonus
(E) cardiorespiratory irregularities

38. All the following statements about the behavioral assessment of alcohol abuse are true EXCEPT

(A) persons with a high degree of acquired tolerance tend to exhibit less evidence of behavioral impairment than those with less tolerance
(B) trained clinical observers are prone to frequent errors when estimating the actual levels of intoxication of alcohol abusers
(C) women attain higher blood levels, absorb alcohol faster, and reach peak blood alcohol levels sooner than men
(D) police officers are more accurate in estimating blood alcohol levels than are social drinkers
(E) in identification of intoxication, the rate of false negative errors is greater than false positive errors

39. When one has no sense of control over a stressful situation, all the following physiologic reactions will occur EXCEPT

(A) weaker corticosteroid elevations will develop
(B) an endogenous opioid peptide will be released
(C) a brief endogenous opiate analgesia will be produced
(D) greater suppression of the cytotoxicity of natural killer cells will occur than in controllable stress
(E) a weaker immune response to mitogen stimulation will develop than in controllable stress

40. In attempting to moderate stress, it has been found that lack of sense of control will result in all the following EXCEPT

(A) increased incidence of gastric ulceration
(B) higher levels of catecholamines if a person's job is self-paced
(C) increased excretion of epinephrine under conditions of uncertainty
(D) comparatively lower levels of corticosteroid production if stress if predictable
(E) lower rate of corticosteroid decline after termination of the stress

41. Metabolic changes occurring during exercise include all the following EXCEPT

(A) the rate of glucose removal from the blood and plasma increases
(B) the amount of insulin required for glucose uptake increases
(C) the sensitivity of insulin receptors in skeletal muscle increases
(D) the sensitivity of insulin receptors in adipose tissue increases
(E) metabolic rate remains elevated for some hours after moderate-to-vigorous exercise

42. Communication between the brain, immune system, and endocrine cells has been confirmed by all the following findings EXCEPT

(A) stimulation of the anterior hypothalamus enhances immune responsivity
(B) high concentrations of peptides are found in the limbic system
(C) immune cells and brain cells produce the same neuropeptides
(D) some brain peptide hormones stimulate T cells to produce lymphokines
(E) the autonomic nervous system controls the immune response

DIRECTIONS: Each group of questions below consists of lettered headings followed by a set of numbered items. For each numbered items select the **one** lettered heading with which it is **most** closely associated. Each lettered heading may be used **once, more than once, or not at all.**

Questions 43–46

For each description that follows, select the substance with which it is most closely associated.

    (A) Dopamine
    (B) Dopamine-β-hydroxylase
    (C) 6-Hydroxydopamine
    (D) Norepinephrine
    (E) Acetylcholine

43. Transmitter that ultimately mediates all overt behavior

44. Substance that poisons neurons by forming peroxides and has been implicated in the cause of schizophrenia

45. Agent that mediates behavioral reward and is found at high levels in the median forebrain bundle

46. Agent that is a putative transmitter and also a precursor of another transmitter in the brain reward system

Questions 47–51

Match the following descriptions with the appropriate stages of sleep.

    (A) Stage 1 REM sleep
    (B) Stage 1 NREM sleep
    (C) Stages 1 through 4 slow wave sleep (NREM)
    (D) Stage 4 delta wave sleep (NREM)
    (E) Stage 2 NREM sleep

47. Decline in heart rate, blood pressure, and respiration and increase in gastrointestinal movements

48. Greatest likelihood of sleeper awakening spontaneously

49. Highest frequency of dream recall

50. Longer duration during the first half of night

51. Continuous decline in the elderly

Questions 52–56

Match the descriptions below with the substances produced by smoking behavior.

(A) Nicotine
(B) Carbon monoxide
(C) Hydrogen cyanide
(D) Both hydrogen cyanide and carbon monoxide
(E) Both nicotine and carbon monoxide

52. Contribution to increased prevalence of fatal and nonfatal cardiovascular disease

53. Promotion of chronic obstructive pulmonary disease, emphysema, and chronic bronchitis

54. Valuable in the discrimination of smokers from nonsmokers

55. Decreased oxygen content in fetal blood and subsequent complications in pregnancy

56. Elevated blood levels from exposure to smoke from other people's cigarettes

Questions 57–60

For each description select the biologic system or substance with which it is most closely associated.

(A) Endocrine and autonomic nervous systems
(B) Hypothalamic-limbic-midbrain circuits
(C) Adrenal cortex and thyroid
(D) Neuropeptides
(E) Dopaminergic circuit or system

57. Highly relevant for Parkinson's disease and schizophrenia

58. Active in mediating integrative processes relevant to survival

59. Substantially involved in mediating adaptive functions of memory appraisal and motivational-emotional response

60. Especially active when one becomes very upset, angry, or depressed for an extended period of time

Questions 61–65

For each psychological response, select the biologic system or anatomic region with which it is most closely associated.

   (A) Sympathoadrenomedullary system
   (B) Hypothalamic-pituitary-adrenocortical (HPAC) system
   (C) Immune system
   (D) Endorphin-enkephalin system
   (E) Anterior hypothalamus

61. Suppressed by stress

62. Increased metabolic activity in response to stress

63. Reduction of fear and pain in aversive situations

64. Implicated in hypertension, angina pectoris, and cardiac arrhythmia

65. Suppressed by increased lympholytic steroid hormones

Questions 66–68

For each behavioral science contribution or concept described, select the person(s) to whom it is attributed.

   (A) Robert Ader
   (B) George Solomon
   (C) Ronald Glaser
   (D) Thomas Holmes and Richard Rahe
   (E) Janis Kiecolt-Glaser

66. Measurement of effects of stress on health

67. Classical conditioning and modulation of immune function

68. Original concept of psychoimmunology

Questions 69–70

For each description, match the appropriate response or pathway.

   (A) Epinephrine and norepinephrine response
   (B) Hypothalamic-pituitary-adrenocortical pathways
   (C) Corticotropin (ACTH) and cortisol pathways
   (D) Sympathoadrenomedullary pathways
   (E) Catecholamine biosynthetic pathways

69. Preferentially active during problem-focused coping

70. Preferentially active during emotion-focused coping

Questions 71–74

For each manifestation described, select the area (zone) in the cerebral cortex with which it is most closely associated.

   (A) Wernicke's area
   (B) Primary sensory/motor areas (ideotypic)
   (C) Unimodal association areas (homotypic)
   (D) Braca's area
   (E) Heteromodal association areas (homotypic)
   (F) Corpus callosum
   (G) Paralimbic areas
   (H) Occipital lobe
   (I) Limbic areas

71. A 47-year-old woman presents with considerable loss of affect and occasional disruption of her memory

72. A 60-year-old male pianist complains that his sense of touch is not as acute and responsive as it used to be

73. A 70-year-old man is hospitalized for a suspected stroke; suddenly he is unable to recognize family or friends

74. A 65-year-old woman has noticed that she is having increased difficulty naming familiar objects, such as a telephone, automobile, or pencil

Questions 75–78

For each concept in behavioral science, select the person to whom it is attributed.

   (A) Alfred Adler
   (B) Harry Stack Sullivan
   (C) George Engel
   (D) Sigmund Freud
   (E) Neal Miller
   (F) René Spitz
   (G) Franz Alexander

75. The biopsychosocial model in medical practice and medical education

76. Instrumental conditioning of autonomically mediated visceral responses

77. Psychological factors that lead to development of specific illnesses

78. Overcoming inferiority through power and mastery

Questions 79–81

For each description, select the neurochemical transmitter with which it is most closely associated.

    (A) Acetylcholine
    (B) Glutamate
    (C) Norepinephrine
    (D) Serotonin
    (E) Dopamine
    (F) Gamma-aminobutyric acid
        (GABA)

79. Plays an important role in the development of depression

80. Has a modulating effect on anxiety

81. Essential for memory

Biologic Correlates
of Behavior
Answers

1.   The answer is C. *(Ader, 2/e, pp 850–858.)* In studying peripheral blood lymphocytes (PBLs) from patients with a major depression, it was found that they had poorer DNA repair (PBLs exposed to radiation damage) than lymphocytes obtained from nondepressed or low-distressed persons. When patients with a diagnosis of major depression were divided into low- and high-distress subgroups, the PBLs from the high-distress subgroup had poorer DNA repair than the PBLs from the low-distress subgroup. While acute stress is immunosuppressive, chronic stress over time is associated with adaptation or even enhancement of immunity. Psychosocial stress and DNA repair in cancer patients have not been studied, although it is hypothesized that the impact of psychosocial stress (distress) on DNA repair could increase cancer risk. The increased anxiety and depression from bereavement does produce suppressed lymphocyte proliferative response to mitogen stimulation 2 to 6 weeks after the death of a spouse. Such impairments of the immune system can be potentially significant in the etiology of cancer.

2.   The answer is D. *(Kandel, 3/e, pp 869–880.)* Clinical studies of patients with major depressive disorders indicate that an intrinsic regulatory defect involving the hypothalamus underlies the disorder. It also involves the monoamine pathways. The hypothalamic modulation of neuroendocrine activity has been implicated, as have been the neurotransmitter systems of serotonin and norepinephrine. Recent evidence suggests a major role for the heritability of such neurochemical disorders. The role of behavior in stimulating or triggering such mechanisms is also being explored. While the frontal lobes, the pituitary, the hippocampus, and the corpus callosum are related to the emotions, memory, and neural communications, they do not play as major a role in the depressive disorders as does the hypothalamus.

3.   The answer is C. *(Kandel, 3/e, pp 217–218, 397–398.)* Under stressful conditions, the organism secretes endorphins and ACTH together. Pro-opiocortin is a common precursor. The close link between endorphins and ACTH suggests that they serve a mediation function for a closely related set of adaptation responses. Thus, they can facilitate one's response to stress and at the same time help one to withstand pain and mobilize for coping activity to deal with the stressful challenge or threat. Almost every physical stress agent increases plasma levels of β-endorphin as well as adrenocorticotropin and corticosterone.

4. The answer is D. *(Carlson, 4/e, pp 273–286.)* More is known about the effects of depriving a person of various kinds of sleep, such as dream sleep, than about the effects of total deprivation of sleep. There appears to be a need for a certain amount of dream sleep. A deficiency produces a "rebound" phenomenon of increased dreaming when uninterrupted sleep is permitted. Contrary to earlier speculations, dream deprivation does not produce any major impairment in psychological functions, nor does it produce any impairment of performance on simple verbal tasks with no emotional content. Dream sleep deprivation, however, does impair the recall of emotionally toned words. It somehow assists the integration of emotional material with memories of other experiences. A major effect of dream deprivation is that it retards formation of memory. An interesting variation is that new learning experiences result in an increase in subsequent dream sleep.

5. The answer is B. *(Isselbacher, 13/e, pp 1366–1373.)* Duodenal ulcer is a chronic and recurrent disease in 6 to 15 percent of the population. It is difficult to establish biologic and behavioral etiologies. It was once thought that it occurred in persons with a unique personality exhibiting oral-receptive characteristics and unmet oral needs, but such a personality has not been substantiated. Chronic anxiety and stress play a major role in the recurrence and exacerbation of ulcer activity. Cigarette smoking and dietary practices (including consumption of alcohol and coffee) can also trigger ulcer activity. Socioeconomic status, occupation, aging, race, and gender have not been identified as factors in frequency of duodenal ulcers.

6. The answer is E. *(Gatchel, 2/e, p 159.)* Traditionally, minor tranquilizers have been used as a standard approach to the treatment of psychophysiologic disorders. Their major defect is that they fail to deal with the underlying psychological, social, or physiologic problem, especially on a long-term basis. They are effective in providing short-term relief for high levels of stress or anxiety and can be more effective if combined with behavior therapy or psychotherapy. Interpersonal dilemmas are not affected, though they may seem to be temporarily dulled with minor tranquilizers. They often have the side effect of drowsiness, can lead to tolerance with the need for increased dosages, and can produce withdrawal symptoms of insomnia, tremors, and even hallucinations.

7. The answer is B. *(Gatchel, 2/e, pp 156–157.)* The diathesis-stress model of psychophysiologic disorders states that individuals are predisposed toward a particular mental or physiologic reaction and that the disorder will become manifest as a reaction to stress. Two major factors are postulated by the model: (1) individual response stereotype, consisting of a predisposition to respond physiologically to various situations and in a particular way; and (2) inadequate homeostatic restraints caused by stress-induced breakdown, previous accident, infection or trauma, or by genetic predisposition. Situational determinants play an important role as does one's perception of the situation, which generates increased or decreased physiologic response. While one's coping style and one's values or attitudes can play a role, they are not considered to be major factors in the diathesis-stress model. The role of learned response can also be important, but is not a major postulate.

8. The answer is C. *(Kaplan, 7/e, pp 43, 162.)* In the late 1950s, Harry Harlow discovered that monkeys reared with a substitute "mother" covered with terry cloth were much more likely to engage in effective heterosexual relationships as juveniles than were monkeys raised with a substitute mother made of steel wire. He concluded that the comfort provided by the clothed (or natural) mother was a critical precursor of the feeling of love. He also demonstrated its importance for positive social and emotional development.

9. The answer is B. *(Carlson, 4/e, pp 357–376.)* In most species, the male tends to be more aggressive than the female. Animal handlers long have taken advantage of the fact that castration, by reducing aggression, makes animals more tractable. Testosterone administered postpubertally to castrated rats can restore aggressiveness to almost normal levels. Similarly, neonatal female mice develop masculine aggressive behavior on receiving androgens. Androgens also promote aggression in humans. Boys are more aggressive than girls at ages 3 to 10, as has been demonstrated in studies of male and female children. Criminals with a history of violence have also been found to have differences in testosterone levels, but it is not yet certain whether the higher androgen levels promote violence or the aggression increases the androgen levels. Probably both mechanisms are active.

10. The answer is C. *(Sierles, p 405.)* A placebo effect is the ability of an inactive substance or condition to induce a therapeutic effect. The therapeutic change is usually positive, but it can also be negative, as can the effect of a chemically active drug. In conditions of pain and anxiety, the greater the pain or anxiety, the greater the placebo effect (contrary to common belief). The placebo effect is thought to be mediated by endogenous opiates stimulated by the brain, which can also play a modulating role in the immune response. Modulated conditioning is not a therapeutic mechanism. Reaction formation is the adoption of attitudes or behaviors that are the opposite of one's real feelings. Fantasy reaction is not related to placebo, which is a real reaction or change. Nonpharmaceutical reaction can be the result of a placebo, but placebo is much broader than a pharmaceutical or nonpharmaceutical reaction.

11. The answer is A. *(Kandel, 3/e, pp 806–810.)* About 30 to 35 percent of the people who cannot sleep have a relatively simple organic cause for the problem. The two most frequent organic causes are disruption of normal circadian rhythms and the inevitable consequences of aging. The most common disruptions of normal circadian rhythms are related to travel, "jet lag," and behavioral changes in one's normal daily routine, such as napping, irregular sleep hours and conditions, alteration in meal times, and unusual work schedules. Normal aging is the next most common factor as it is more difficult to reset one's biologic clock the older one gets. It has been estimated that most people over age 60 sleep only about 5.5 h per day, and since stage 4 NREM sleep also declines with age, the lighter stages of NREM sleep allow the person to awaken more often, sometimes generating the worry that one cannot sleep or that one is not getting enough sleep. Accumulation of hepatic enzymes is a frequent side effect of prolonged use of sleeping pills. The most common psychosocial cause of insomnia is emotional disturbance.

12. The answer is B. *(Kandel, 3/e, pp 1027–1030.)* The relationship between social and biologic processes has historically been regarded by psychiatry and medicine as organic and functional. Organic mental illnesses have included the dementias and the toxic psychoses. The functional mental illnesses have included the various depressive syndromes, the schizophrenias, and the neuroses. When anatomic evidence of brain lesions was produced, the diseases were called *organic*, and those that lacked these features were labeled *functional*. This distinction should be considered artificial and historical since organic and functional diseases affect mentation and vice versa. In fact, all mental processes are biologic and any alteration of these processes is organic. The most significant questions to ask about disease or behavior concern the degree to which a biologic or behavioral process is determined by genetic and developmental factors versus toxic or infectious agents versus environmental, social, or behavioral determinants. Psychoanalytic (dynamic) approaches and an understanding of conditioning (learning) played important roles in the evolution and development of a more integrated biobehavioral understanding of human behavior and human biology.

13. The answer is D. *(Feuerstein, pp 220–221.)* The use of relaxation techniques to reduce stress has proved very effective. Studies of diabetic patients who practiced progressive muscle relaxation showed significant improvement in glucose tolerance following relaxation training. Plasma cortisol levels were also reduced in patients trained in relaxation. Relaxation, however, did not affect insulin sensitivity or glucose-stimulated secretion of insulin. Stress reduction techniques, such as relaxation, are effective in reducing requirements for exogenous insulin and in the management of both insulin-dependent and non-insulin-dependent diabetes.

14. The answer is A. *(Kandel, 3/e, pp 653–654.) Paradoxical sleep* is a term given to REM sleep, which is considered paradoxical because its electroencephalographic pattern resembles that of the alert waking state. Dreaming occurs during REM sleep. When a person is repeatedly awakened during dreaming, a dream deprivation occurs and there is a rebound phenomenon of increased frequency and lengthening of dreaming when the person is permitted to sleep normally. Dream deprivation does not result in a major decrement in psychological or intellectual functions (as does sleep deprivation), but it does appear to retard the memory formation of emotionally toned words. While earlier studies suggested the presence of bizarre behavior, anxiety, irritability, and nightmares, more recent studies have found no such changes in humans even after 16 days of deprivation of dream sleep.

15. The answer is B. *(Rosen, pp 305–306.)* Of the immunologic components that interact with tumor cells, such as T lymphocytes, macrophages, and humoral antibodies, the natural killer cells show a decrease in activity after psychosocial stress; the most active mechanism is corticosteroid production through the hypothalamic-pituitary-adrenal axis. Natural killer cells play a role in the inhibition of tumor growth and in the surveillance against newly developing primary tumors, at distant sites as well as locally in the body. Recent studies by Glaser, Kiecolt-Glaser, Schleifer, Keller, and others have linked the activity of natural killer cells to examination stress, vulnerability to viruses, depression, infectious illness, and bereavement.

16. The answer is C. *(Sierles, pp 400–402.)* During active coping (Cannon's fight-or-flight) there is an increase in heart rate, cardiac output, activity of striate muscle, catecholamines, and cortisol, along with vasodilation in the muscles. Under the condition of coping effort without distress, there is an increase in catecholamines (especially norepinephrine), but with a suppression of cortisol. On the other hand, coping effort associated with negative emotions (e.g., embarrassment or feeling harassed) leads to preferential secretion of epinephrine. Attempts to cope with such stressful situations over a long period of time has important implications for health maintenance and vulnerability to disease.

17. The answer is C. *(Gatchel, 2/e, pp 18–20.)* Most glands receive either direct neural control from the brain or indirect control from hormones secreted by the hypothalamus. Thus, thyroid secretion is subject to hypothalamic control, whereas insulin secretion depends in part on adrenergic influence from the autonomic nervous system. The parathyroids are notably free of brain control; in regulating calcium metabolism, they in turn are regulated by blood levels of calcium.

18. The answer is B. *(Carlson, 4/e, pp 320–338.)* Oxytocin is one of the peptide hormones that apparently is behaviorally inactive. It has an important function in parturition by facilitating contractions of the uterus; the hormone also facilitates ejection of milk during lactation. The gonadal steroids, in contrast, exert profound effects on behavior. They are necessary for appropriate reproductive and parental behavior patterns in any species of mammals. In addition, gonadal hormones mediate many forms of agonistic behavior.

19. The answer is D. *(Gatchel, 2/e, pp 146–152.)* Psychophysiologic disorders were formerly referred to as *psychosomatic illnesses*. They are characterized by physical symptoms from organs of the body that have become dysfunctional through an interaction between psychological, biologic (including genetic), and sociocultural factors. Specifically, the most common psychophysiologic disorders are bronchial asthma, dysmenorrhea, headache, neurodermatitis, and peptic ulcer. Diabetes, along with many other diseases, has a strong psychological component, but is not considered to be a psychophysiologic disorder.

20. The answer is B. *(Kandel, 3/e, pp 258–262.)* When the axon is cut, the axon and synaptic terminals are deprived of essential metabolic connections with the cell body. Since axonal transport occurs in both directions, the result is a rapid local degeneration of the axon and myelin sheath, with the cell body also being affected. Synapses mediate both electrical signals and nutritive interactions between neurons. Thus, changes occur in the cell body (retrograde changes) and also in subsequent neurons that receive synapses from the damaged neurons. Macrophages from the general circulation enter the trauma area and phagocytose axonal debris, and glial cells (astrocytes and microglia) proliferate to assist in the process. This proliferation of fibrous astrocytes forms a glial scar around the trauma area, which can then block the course of regenerating axons and the reformation of central connections. The behavioral effects of nerve lesions are peculiar to the location of the lesion in the brain and the nerve cell connections, so that the same type of injury will have different behavioral effects depending on its location.

21. The answer is B. *(Gatchel, 2/e, pp 121–126.)* *Immunocompetence* refers to the ability of the various components of the immune system to recognize, respond to, and reject elements and antigens that do not belong in the body. The immune system can no longer be regarded as an autonomous system. The autonomic and central nervous systems and the endocrine system have been known to influence and to be influenced by the immune system, and it has now been demonstrated that psychosocial factors can also influence the immune system and affect its ability to respond to invading organisms and antigens. Psychosocial stress can suppress immunocompetence. While acute stress tends to suppress the immune system, chronic stress tends to enhance the immune system, especially over time.

22. The answer is C. *(Kandel, 3/e, pp 945–957.)* All functions of the brain represent an interaction between genetic and environmental factors (e.g., learning). It is also known that the structure of the brain is greatly influenced by genetic and developmental processes. It is not always appreciated that the structure of the brain, specifically the pattern of interconnections between the neurons, also depends on experience with behavior. This influence is established early, in that there are certain critical stages in the development of the brain when the integrative action of the brain and its cellular structure are dependent upon its interaction with its environment. Further, the work of Harry Harlow with isolated young monkeys, the work of René Spitz and others with early human sensory and social deprivation, and the early sensory deprivation perception studies of von Senden, Riesen, Hubel, and Wiesel have soundly established the importance of the critical period concept upon the development of normal social behavior, physical growth, and normal visual perception. The influence and the action of the environment on the brain do vary with age— both normal and abnormal patterns of stimulation have a more profound effect at early stages of development. Environmental stimuli, social experience, and learning and memory also continue to have an influence on adults.

23. The answer is A. *(Gatchel, 2/e, pp 128–129.)* The immune system may control latent viruses such as Epstein-Barr or herpes simplex, but it cannot destroy or eliminate them. If the immune system is weakened so that the virus becomes more active, the antibody titers to the virus will increase. Immunosuppressive drugs will increase antibodies to latent viruses. Kiecolt-Glaser and Glaser, working with medical students and elderly residents of nursing homes, were able to demonstrate that the stress of examinations and loneliness were associated with elevated antibody titers. Sustained noise also causes a rise in antibody titers initially, but after a few days the organism seems to adapt and titers return to normal. Studies have also demonstrated that relaxation training produces decreased antibody titers to latent viruses by generating an increase in natural killer cell activity.

24. The answer is D. *(Lindzey, 3/e, pp 855–859.)* The secretion of epinephrine and norepinephrine (catecholamines), which is accelerated under conditions of psychosocial stress, induces pathogenic states leading to cardiovascular disease—for example, increased blood pressure and heart rate, elevated blood lipids, acceleration of the rate of damage to the inner areas of the coronary arteries, and also the induction or provocation of ventricular arrhythmias. First-degree AV block is a conduction disorder unrelated to stress. The provocation of ventricular arrhythmias is especially important as a potential cause of sudden death.

25. The answer is E. *(Lindzey, 3/e, pp 859–860.)* If a person is agitated, anxious, in a state of panic or near panic, or in a state of hypervigilance to minor or major threat cues, increased breathing (hyperventilation) is a frequent response. Typically, a series of major physiologic, behavioral, and psychological changes is evoked. The reduced CO_2 in the blood lowers the blood's acid level; sympathetic activity, cardiac arrhythmias, and heart rate increase; decreased oxygen is supplied to brain tissue; and cerebral vasoconstriction is heightened. Acute anxiety ensues, generally focused on the threatening situation or somatic complaints, and the sense of fear is heightened. The altered patterns of vascular, neurologic, and cerebral activity are mainly responsible for the psychomotor and cognitive impairments. Such psychological, social, physical, or environmental hypervigilance frequently results in temporary impairment and defective decision-making characterized by excessive vacillation and an impulsive choice of options.

26. The answer is D. *(Ader, 2/e, pp 850–864. Gatchel, 2/e, pp 125–133.)* A number of experimental and clinical studies on the effects of psychosocial stress on the human immune system have demonstrated a decrease in the activity of natural killer cells in healthy human subjects. Likewise, stress was related to a decrease in lymphocyte cytotoxicity and a decrease in the rate of microbe engulfment by polymorphonuclear granulocytes. There was also a depression in the response of T lymphocytes to mitogens. Latent viruses, such as herpes simplex or Epstein-Barr, are generally controlled by the immune system, but when the immune system is suppressed, the antibody titers to the virus will increase. Another study demonstrated that sleep deprivation decreased the ability of blood neutrophil granulocytes to phagocytize *Staphylococcus aureus* and increased the production of interferon by blood lymphocytes. Also, the phytohemagglutinin-induced DNA synthesis of blood lymphocytes was reduced after sleep deprivation of 48 h.

27. The answer is E. *(Rosen, pp 114–116.)* Vigorous exercise over time has been shown to increase the high-density lipoprotein cholesterol in the blood while decreasing the low-density lipoprotein cholesterol, very low-density lipoprotein cholesterol, total cholesterol, and triglycerides. Thus, vigorous exercise acts to reduce several established risk factors for coronary heart disease and to promote increased high-density lipoprotein cholesterol, which has an antiatherogenic effect.

28. The answer is B. *(Kandel, 3/e, pp 7–10.)* While the control of certain intellectual functions by the right hemisphere or left hemisphere is not as clear-cut and clearly divided as was once thought, there are still general functions related to the right or left hemisphere. The left hemisphere is much more involved in language, smaller muscle movements, vocalization, finger dexterity, and logic. The right is much more involved in large motor programs, great muscles of the limbs, spatial abilities, and "gestalt" thinking. It is important to remember that the hemispheres do interact with each other.

29. The answer is E. *(Williams, RB, pp 3–9.)* Research on hypothalamic hormones has led to the discovery of many neuropeptides. The study of endorphins that bind to various opiate receptors in the brain has led to some amazing discoveries. Dynorphin, a natural brain endorphin, is reported to be 200 times more potent than morphine and 50 times more potent than other known endorphins. The high degree of potency indicates that it is able to bind with great specificity to pain receptors, but it also appears to produce tolerance and dependence. While it is highly potent, it is still experimental and not in clinical use. It occurs in the pituitary, other parts of the brain, spinal cord, and adrenal medulla.

30. The answer is A. *(Sierles, pp 185–187.)* Many psychiatric disorders manifest evidence of brain dysfunction. Evidence of such brain dysfunction has been found in 50 percent or more of patients with schizophrenia. For example, a neurologic examination will demonstrate soft signs (e.g., grasp reflex, rooting reflex, motor impersistence) in 70 percent of adult schizophrenics; 75 percent (whether ill or recovered) will also demonstrate abnormalities in eye pursuit; 75 percent will have moderate-to-severe bilateral impairment on neuropsychological tests; and 50 percent will have nonspecific abnormalities on the EEG. Also, 50 percent will have some cortical atrophy and ventricular enlargement on imaging tests. The lactate infusion test induces panic behavior in 80 percent of patients with panic disorder, but not in patients with schizophrenia.

31. The answer is D. *(Gatchel, 2/e, p 133.)* Consumption of alcohol has been shown to affect the immune system, apparently in relation to dose. Macrophages are inhibited and move more slowly toward chemical signals released by the body. Proliferation and cytotoxicity of T cells are also inhibited. Increased doses of alcohol can damage certain bodily tissues, such as the thymus. However, no inhibition of production of antibodies has been observed.

32. The answer is B. *(Kaplan, 7/e, pp 699–703.)* Sleep is divided into two distinct states: D sleep (desynchronized EEG pattern sleep) and S sleep (synchronized EEG pattern sleep). D sleep is also known as REM (rapid eye movement) or dreaming sleep; S sleep as NREM (non-rapid eye movement), orthodox, or quiet sleep. S sleep (NREM) is divided into stages 1, 2, 3, and 4; stage 1 is the lightest and stage 4 the deepest. NREM sleep lasts from 60 to 100 min, followed by 10 to 40 min of REM sleep, and the cycle is continued throughout the night. Typically, about 80 percent of an adult's sleep time is spent in NREM sleep and 20 percent in REM sleep. REM sleep tends to increase during the second half of the night. The amount of REM sleep appears to determine the amount of rest. When REM sleep is interrupted, tiredness tends to develop. A newborn spends about 50 percent of sleep time in REM sleep. Deep sleep begins to be replaced by longer periods of lighter sleep after the age of 30.

33. The answer is B. *(Kandel, 3/e, pp 258–262.)* The cutting of a nerve tract within the brain or of a peripheral nerve results in the following sequence: Both ends of the cut axon immediately seal off the axoplasm, retract, and begin to swell; there is rapid degeneration of the axon and the myelin sheath; the macrophages from the general circulation enter the area and phagocytose axonal debris; there is also a proliferation of glial cells, which act as phagocytes; and fibrous astrocytes proliferate in the central nervous system, which leads to glial scar formation around the zone of trauma that often blocks the course taken by regenerating axons and causes a barrier against the reformation of central connections. Degeneration spreads along the axon in both directions from the zone of trauma. The retrograde reaction in the proximal segment usually progresses a short distance and appears in the cell body after 2 to 3 days. In the distal segment, degeneration appears in the axon terminal in about 1 day, and within 2 weeks the distal synapses degenerate completely.

34. The answer is E. *(Sierles, pp 400–402.)* Different kinds of stressors elicit different physiologic responses. Vigilant inaction is a condition in which one is facing stressors for which there is no apparent coping strategy or opportunity for defense. In that case there is increased blood pressure and peripheral blood flow resistance, vagus nerve–mediated bradycardia, decreased cardiac output, increased secretion of corticotropin (ACTH) and cortisol, and decreased levels of brain norepinephrine. When active coping is pursued or becomes an option, adrenal medullary secretion of epinephrine and hypothalamic-pituitary-adrenocortical activity decrease.

35. The answer is B. *(Sierles, pp 393–397.)* Side effects on sexual function are frequently produced by antihypertensives, other cardiovascular compounds, and psychotropic medications. Sexual dysfunctions can be produced through anti-cholinergic parasympathetic and sympathetic ganglionic-blocking, antiandrogenic, beta-adrenergic, progestational, antihistaminic, and dopamine antagonist actions. Tricyclics, phenothiazines, alpha-methyldopa, and guanethidine all have the effect of decreasing sexual arousal. They can also inhibit desire and produce orgasmic difficulties. Amphetamines can produce orgasmic difficulties, but do not appear to inhibit desire or decrease arousal. The physician must always bear in mind that drug combinations can create untoward effects on sexual function.

36. The answer is D. *(Kandel, 3/e, pp 808–810.)* Even though many sleeping pills are initially helpful, they lose their effectiveness within 2 weeks. The repeated administration of barbiturates (e.g., pentobarbital or phenobarbital) results in a gradual increase in hepatic enzymes, which normally are responsible for the degradation of the barbiturates. Not only is their pharmacologic action decreased, but since the liver enzymes are relatively nonspecific, the result is often a broad cross-tolerance to other hypnotics. Barbiturates are known to suppress REM sleep, so that when the drug is withdrawn, a marked REM rebound results, often aggravating insomnia. Even though the benzodiazepines are also addictive, flurazepam increases hepatic enzymes at a much slower rate; hence patients develop a tolerance much more slowly than for pentobarbital. However, an active metabolite of flurazepam remains in the body for a longer period of time (more than 24 h), which results in a gradual increase of these breakdown substances in the blood. Thus, the effects of the drug are often felt during the daytime as diminished alertness and hand-eye coordination. These symptoms are also aggravated by alcohol.

37. The answer is B. *(Kandel, 3/e, pp 795–799.)* The physiologic responses to dreaming listed in the question can easily be recorded in most people several times each night. If awakened at such times, people usually confirm that they were dreaming. This complex of physiologic signs (e.g., electroencephalographic desynchrony, rapid eye movements, loss of muscle tonus, and cardiorespiratory irregularities) is commonly referred to as *REM (rapid eye movement) sleep* or *paradoxical sleep*. The term *paradoxical sleep* was applied originally because the associated electroencephalographic pattern is characteristic of the alert waking state despite the fact that the dreaming person is, in fact, sound asleep. Dreams occurring during non-REM sleep are less easily recalled, less vivid, less visual, less emotional, and more pleasant.

38. The answer is D. *(Schneiderman, pp 379–399.)* It has been demonstrated that persons with a high degree of acquired tolerance are less apt to evidence impairments or exhibit overt signs of intoxication than those who drink "socially." Some tolerant persons can perform psychomotor skills and good mentation with blood alcohol levels between 200 and 300 mg percent. Also, estimates of intoxication based on observations of a drinker's behavior are apt to be invalid. Studies have shown that even trained clinical observers and law enforcement officers make frequent errors in estimating actual levels of intoxication of alcohol abusers. The rate of false positive errors (i.e., the identification of a sober person as intoxicated) ranged from 0 to 16.7 percent, while false negative errors (i.e., failure to identify persons with positive blood alcohol levels) ranged from 22.2 to 55 percent. Thus, the accuracy of estimates of blood alcohol is extremely variable, with most officers no more accurate than a similarly tested group of social drinkers. Women are more responsive than men to the same dose of alcohol, apparently as a function of hormonal level and stage in the menstrual cycle. Women attain higher blood levels, absorb alcohol faster, and reach peak blood alcohol levels sooner than men; women are even more responsive the day preceding the menstrual cycle and about the time of ovulation.

39. The answer is A. *(Gatchel, 2/e, pp 78–79.)* Stress without the sense of control has been found to influence the release of endogenous opioid peptides, such as β-endorphin. When one learns that one has no control over a stressful situation, an opiate-based analgesia occurs. Both uncontrollable and controllable stressors produce a brief poststressor analgesia, but only the opioid produced by inescapable stressors can be blocked by administering opiate antagonists. Both controllable and uncontrollable stress situations suppress the cytotoxicity of natural killer cells, but inescapable and uncontrollable stress results in greater suppression than does controllable and escapable stress. Corticosteroid release during uncontrollable or inescapable stress is somewhat greater than when the stress can be controlled or escaped. Corticosteroid levels also decline more slowly after uncontrollable stress.

40. The answer is B. *(Gatchel, 2/e, pp 77–79.)* Having some sense of control over a stressful situation is an important factor in coping with stress and reducing the physiologic reactions to stress. In situations that are uncontrollable, unpredictable, inescapable, or uncertain, the levels of corticosteroids and catecholamines are increased. Furthermore, corticosteroid levels decline more slowly after the termination of an uncontrollable or inescapable stress. Unpredictable shock with no control has also produced an increased incidence of gastric ulceration in animals. In stressful occupational situations, those workers whose jobs are self-paced show fewer symptoms of stress and less catecholamine excretion than those whose jobs are machine-paced. Thus, the potential danger of sustained higher levels of physiologic reactions to stress is reduced by the person's having some level of control. Situations involving uncertainty also involve an increase in the excretion of epinephrine, norepinephrine, and cortisol.

41. The answer is B. *(Rosen, pp 116–117.)* It has been recognized that exercise decreases the symptoms of hyperglycemia. Under conditions of oral glucose challenge or glucose infusion into the blood stream, physically active persons have an increased rate of glucose removal and a decreased amount of insulin required. Also, the insulin receptors in skeletal muscle and adipose tissue show an increase in sensitivity. Thus, carbohydrate metabolism improves with exercise and physical activity and, within limits, appears to improve with the intensity and duration of the exercise. In addition, the metabolic rate will remain elevated for some hours after moderate-to-vigorous exercise.

42. The answer is E. *(Sierles, pp 404–405.)* The brain and endocrine and immune systems communicate with and influence each other. Studies of the hypothalamus have demonstrated that stimulation of the anterior hypothalamus enhances immune responsiveness, and stimulation of the posterior lobe inhibits immune reactivity. Removal of the thymus gland will result in the atrophy of these hypothalamic neurons. Also, the limbic system contains high concentrations of neuropeptide receptors, as do the lining of the intestines and lymphocytes. It has also been found that immune cells produce the same neuropeptides that are produced in the brain. Some of these peptide hormones that are produced in the brain stimulate T cells to produce lymphokines, such as interleukins and interferon. Historically, the immune system was thought to be a more or less autonomous system that involved only the autonomic nervous system (ANS), but with the demonstration of the "hard wiring" connections of the immune system with the central nervous system and of neural, endocrine, and behavioral interactions, the ANS is now considered to be only one of the interacting and collaborating systems.

43–46. The answers are 43-E, 44-C, 45-D, 46-A. *(Carlson, 4/e, pp 47–72.)* Acetylcholine is the transmitter agent at the neuromuscular junction. It is released from presynaptic neuron terminals in quantal amounts and excites contractile mechanisms in postsynaptic muscle fibers. Since muscular contractions are the substrate of all behavior patterns, it may be said that acetylcholine is the ultimate mediator of all behavior.

The enzyme dopamine-β-hydroxylase catalyzes the conversion of dopamine to norepinephrine. Evidence suggests that the brains of schizophrenic persons may be deficient in this important enzyme. It is unclear whether this psychopathology results from an accumulation of dopamine or from a relative lack of norepinephrine.

Schizophrenia may result in part from the presence of 6-hydroxydopamine in the brain. This substance destroys noradrenergic terminals because of its tendency to form toxic peroxides. In theory, an inborn error of metabolism could produce a high cerebral concentration of 6-hydroxydopamine. Schizophrenia would then occur because of disturbed function in the noradrenergic terminal fields of the brain.

The brain structure most effective in producing positive reinforcement of operant behavior from electric stimulation is the median forebrain bundle. This structure is closely related anatomically and physiologically to the lateral hypothalamic nucleus. The median forebrain bundle contains very high levels of norepinephrine. Apparently, as a neurotransmitter norepinephrine is involved in mediating behavioral reward and motivational processes.

Both dopamine and norepinephrine are capable of functioning as neurotransmitters. Norepinephrine is formed from dopamine in the presence of dopamine-β-hydroxylase. Insofar as norepinephrine may be involved in behavioral reward, its precursor, dopamine, also would be involved.

47–51. The answers are 47-C, 48-A, 49-A, 50-D, 51-D. *(Kandel, 3/e, pp 792–803.)* Sleep is a rhythmic and active neural and behavioral process. The sleep-wake cycle is an endogenous rhythm of the body (as are such rhythms as body temperature, urine formation, and cortisol secretion). Human sleep varies from five to seven orderly cycles each night and is characterized by stages 1 through 4 (with increasing slow wave NREM sleep) occurring in the first 30 to 45 min, stage 4 being the deepest sleep; the EEG shows that the same stages are then retraced in reverse order. As the stages or depths of sleep increase, the autonomic indicators demonstrate a parasympathetic dominance, with heart rate, blood pressure, and respiration declining and becoming more even, and gastrointestinal mobility increasing. The sleeper is more apt to be awakened spontaneously in stage 1 REM sleep than in stage 4 REM sleep.

Stage 1 REM (rapid eye movement) sleep is distinguishable from stage 1 NREM (non–rapid eye movement) sleep by additional electrooculographic and electromyographic criteria. Stage 1 REM sleep is considered to be the dream phase. The first REM sleep period is usually short (5 to 10 min) but tends to increase with each successive sleep cycle. Stages 3 and 4 NREM sleep dominate during the first third or half of the night and are less frequent during the later or early morning cycles. Dreams are recalled best when one is awakened from stage 1 REM sleep and less well during subsequent deeper NREM stages of sleep.

Stage 4 NREM sleep decreases with age and sometimes disappears in persons over 60 years of age. This continuous decline in the elderly is correlated with an increase in the number of spontaneous awakenings. REM sleep and stage 4 NREM sleep are differentially affected by certain psychoactive drugs, especially alcohol and barbiturates, which suppress REM sleep, while stage 4 NREM sleep is especially decreased by the benzodiazepines diazepam (Valium) and chlordiazepoxide (Librium).

Stage 2 NREM sleep increases toward the end of the sleep period and occupies about half of the total sleep time. Dream recall is less if one is awakened during stage 2 NREM sleep than if awakened during stage 1 NREM or stage 1 REM sleep.

52–56. The answers are 52-E, 53-C, 54-C, 55-B, 56-B. *(Gatchel, 2/e, pp 281–289.)* Carbon monoxide produced by smoking behavior is a major health hazard for smokers and nonsmokers. Elevated levels play a role in the etiology of most cardiovascular diseases, including coronary heart disease. It has been associated with peripheral vascular disease, reduced cardiac output, and reduced duration of exercise prior to angina. It also results in decreased oxygen content of fetal blood in a pregnancy as well as subsequent complications in pregnancy. The combination of carbon monoxide and nicotine in smokers contributes to the increased prevalence of fatal and nonfatal cardiovascular disease.

Even though cigarette smoking is by far the major source of exposure to carbon monoxide, occupational exposure (e.g., in blast furnace workers, automobile mechanics, traffic control officers, taxi drivers, truck drivers) as well as urban living and exposure to other people's cigarette smoke can lead to elevated carbon monoxide levels, often with concentrations as high as those of smokers. Other factors affecting one's carbon monoxide level include individual response variability, the way a cigarette is smoked, rate of consumption, the smoker's activity levels, and the variety of tobacco product being smoked. Alcohol consumption will also affect carbon monoxide levels.

Hydrogen cyanide gas is a constituent of cigarette smoke and a primary ciliatoxic agent in cigarette smoking. It is implicated in the development of chronic obstructive pulmonary disease, emphysema, and chronic bronchitis. The combination of hydrogen cyanide gas and carbon monoxide is also implicated in the development of atherosclerosis. Measurement of thiocyanate, the primary metabolite of hydrogen cyanide, serves as an excellent index of smoking behavior and it is also valuable in the discrimination of smokers from non-smokers. Thiocyanate is also associated with stomach cancer.

Nicotine is inhaled with each puff of cigarette smoke and is now regarded as the major pharmacologic addicting agent in smoking. It is absorbed from the lungs so quickly that in only 5 min it can be found in the brain, adrenal medulla, and sympathetic ganglia. Most persons smoke to obtain pharmacologically satisfying doses of nicotine, and they become so accustomed to certain levels of nicotine that they maintain these levels by titrating nicotine intake and adjusting their smoking behavior accordingly. Even though it has central nervous system and cocarcinogenic effects, it primarily acts upon the cardiovascular and respiratory systems. Its deleterious actions on the cardiovascular system include a hemodynamic response of increased work for the heart, increased circulation of fatty acids, and an increase in platelet adhesion and aggregation. While nicotine increases the amount of work of the heart, carbon monoxide reduces the amount of oxygen available to the heart muscle; thus, the combination of carbon monoxide and nicotine links smoking behavior with an increased incidence of atherosclerosis and thrombosis.

57–60. The answers are 57-E, 58-B, 59-B, 60-C. *(Williams, RB, pp 3–9, 25–29.)* One of the major advances of recent research has been the revelation of the brain's strong regulatory influence on the endocrine and autonomic nervous systems. This is most relevant when the organism is exposed to changes in its environmental conditions. The more severe the changes, the more severe the stress. The transmission of information in the brain and between the brain and other tissues and systems involves about a dozen amino acids and monoamines. These neurotransmitters function either at the level of the synapse, or as modulators of information flow between neurons. The best-documented neurotransmitters are dopamine, norepinephrine, serotonin, and gamma-aminobutyric acid.

Each neurotransmitter is differentially distributed in the brain for transmission of information from cell to cell. One such system is the dopaminergic circuit or system. Parkinson's disease is strongly related to the dopaminergic system. The dopaminergic system is also related to schizophrenia.

The hypothalamic-limbic-midbrain circuits exert a strong regulatory influence on both the endocrine system and the autonomic nervous system. As such, these circuits have a major influence on the cardiovascular and gastrointestinal systems. They also play a major role in mediating the adaptive functions of memory, appraisal, and motivational-emotional responses. Thus, the human neocortex is able to mobilize a metabolic and cardiovascular adaptive response for action by first using these circuits to appraise the functional significance of the environment or of ongoing events. By the brain's maintaining a constant reappraisal from ongoing feedback, these hypothalamic-limbic-midbrain circuits are able to mediate the integrative processes relevant to action or survival.

These circuits are also influenced by neuropeptides (e.g., endorphins, enkephalins, vasopressin). Neuropeptides exist as neurotransmitters and as hormones. By clinging to the nerve cell membrane for varying periods of time, they can modulate the flow of information. Thus, it is believed that the neuropeptides may be able to "fine tune" one's mood.

Psychological stress influences the adrenal cortex and the thyroid. These functional changes occur when one is very upset, anxious, angry, or depressed for a long period of time. In effect, all glands controlled by the anterior pituitary are influenced by a stressful experience.

The hypothalamic hormones influence and coordinate the endocrine system and the autonomic nervous system. They are known as the coordinators of coordinators, since the endocrine system and autonomic nervous system each has major coordinating functions.

61–65. The answers are 61-C, 62-A, 63-D, 64-A, 65-C. *(Feuerstein, pp 114–117, 188–189.)* The sympathoadrenomedullary system increases metabolic activity in response to stressful situations. It generally involves physical exertion. The activity of the sympathoadrenomedullarry system is typically measured by norepinephrine and epinephrine. The system is implicated in such physical disorders as hypertension, atherosclerosis, angina pectoris, cardiac arrhythmias, and myocardial ischemia.

The hypothalamic-pituitary-adrenocortical (HPAC) system responds to emotionally stressful situations in which active coping may not be possible. It also responds to heat, cold, infection, sympathomimetic drugs, and surgery. The system is associated with a "conservation-withdrawal" pattern, characterized by such activities as vigilance, sympathetic nervous system activation, inhibition of movement, and bradycardia associated with the parasympathetic nervous system. Less associated with the "conservation-withdrawal" pattern are various cardiovascular diseases, peptic ulceration, suppression of the immune system, and clinical depression.

The immune system is one of several physiologic systems affected by active and passive attempts to cope with stress. Acute stress increases the steroid hormones that are known to be lympholytic, and this response suppresses the immune system. A suppressed immune system increases susceptibility to infection and tumor growth. The immune system is affected by the hypothalamic-pituitary-adrenocortical and central nervous systems.

The endorphin-enkephalin system is involved in aversive situations requiring active coping. It helps reduce fear, inhibit pain-related withdrawal behaviors, and reduce pain during coping responses. These endogenous opiates provide another way for measuring the physiologic components of stress.

When stimulated the anterior hypothalamus elicits the relaxation response. Its counterpart, the posterior area of the hypothalamus, stimulates the fight-or-flight reaction. The relaxation response results in hypo- or adynamia of skeletal musculature, decreased blood pressure, decreased respiratory rate, and constricted pupils. These physiologic changes are consistent with a generalized decrease in sympathetic activity and are different from changes recorded during quiet sitting or sleep.

66–68. The answers are 66-D, 67-A, 68-B. *(Ader, 2/e, pp 852–854. Sierles, pp 400–407.)* Robert Ader, a psychologist, discovered that the immune system can be suppressed through classical conditioning. When he conditioned infected rats to avoid immunity-suppressing and nausea-producing cyclophosphamide as the unconditioned stimulus, he found that the rats continued to die from the infection, even after he stopped giving them cyclophosphamide in the saccharine-flavored water. The immune system had become conditioned to the suppressant effects of the drug. When he used this same protocol with a strain of rats susceptible to an autoimmune disease similar to lupus erythematosus (LE) he found that they had learned to suppress their immune system, thus retarding the autoimmune process, and lived longer than the LE rats. Subsequent experiments established that the human immune system can also be behaviorally conditioned, thus demonstrating the modulating effect of behavior on the immune system through the central nervous system.

George Solomon, an eminent psychiatrist, coined the term *psychoimmunology* in 1964. His published paper with Ruddy Moos (a psychologist)— "Emotions, Immunity, and Disease: A Speculative Theoretical Integration"— was far ahead of its time. Solomon also studied coping activities of AIDS patients and found that those who were more involved in coping activities and who actively participated in their medical care and exercise program had a longer survival time.

Thomas Holmes and Richard Rahe developed a questionnaire to quantify the stress effects of life change and the subsequent development of numerous illnesses. The death of a spouse was a high stressor, while changing a residence was considered relatively low. Even higher levels of positive correlations between life stress events and illness have been achieved by taking into account the meaning and perception of the life event. In general, negative events, such as losses, are more stressful than positive events, and the higher the stressful life change/event, the greater the likelihood of the development of an illness.

Ronald Glaser (a microbiologist and psychoneuroimmunologist) provided molecular biological documentation that stress and distress significantly suppress the process of cellular DNA repair. He found (working with rats) that under conditions of rotational stress, there was a depression of the ability of splenic lymphocytes to synthesize O^6-methylguanine DNA methyltransferase, which is an essential enzyme in the metabolic pathway of DNA repair. This has helped document the crucial importance of recognizing the interaction between psychosocial stress, modulation of DNA repair, and the potential increased risk for the development of abnormal cells or the lack of immunologic protection from such cells.

Janis Kiecolt-Glaser (a psychologist) made some major initial contributions by studying the influence of psychosocial factors (stress) on the immune system of medical students before and after examination time. She then showed that medical students with the most suppression of immune function scored highest on loneliness. Psychiatric inpatients who scored high on loneliness had poorer mitogenic responses. She also documented that caretakers of patients with Alzheimer's disease had to endure severe stress and loneliness, which resulted in poorer cellular immune function than that of controls.

69–70. The answers are 69-D, 70-B. *(Sierles, pp 400–402.)* Potential stressors are evaluated through a process called *cognitive appraisal,* and on the basis of this appraisal, a coping strategy is determined—either one that is problem-focused or one that is emotion-focused. Either may be adaptive or maladaptive, and it is possible for them to occur in combination at various proportions. Problem-focused coping attempts to manage, alter, or take some action to relieve the stressor. Different kinds of stressors and coping responses elicit different autonomic responses. It is now known that the physiologic response to threat is a very complex interaction, and that the sympatho-adrenomedullary (SAM) system is preferentially active during problem-focused coping. Learning and conditioning also play important roles in the process of cognitive appraisal.

In emotion-focused coping, the effort is directed at regulating the emotional response to the threat or problem. This is especially active when the threat or stress cannot be averted. Examples of emotion-focused coping are denial, avoidance, or minimalizing. These responses may be adaptive, e.g., they may facilitate recovery and reduce complications during and after a myocardial infarction, but they may be maladaptive before and after hospitalization. During emotion-focused coping, the hypothalamic-pituitary-adrenocortical (HPAC) system is preferentially active.

Epinephrine and norepinephrine responses, corticotropin and cortisol pathways, and catecholamine biosynthetic pathways are all involved in stress and coping responses in various ways, but are not preferentially active during problem-focused or emotion-focused coping.

71–74. The answers are 71-I, 72-B, 73-C, 74-E. *(Sierles, pp 33–46.)* The limbic area includes the septum pellucidum and septal nuclei, the amygdaloid complex and its nuclei, the hippocampus, and the olfactory tubercle, bulb, and striae. Its main function relates to control over the internal milieu, the modulation of instincts and drives, memory, and learning, and the emotional and affective coloring of experiences. Since the limbic system modulates the formation of everyday affective experiences (e.g., feelings, emotions, and moods), it is important to recognize that diseases or disorders of the limbic system can cause mood disorders and other psychopathology. Influenza epidemics and viral infections of the limbic system have resulted in various psychopathologies such as obsessive-compulsive, manic-depressive, and schizophrenia-like states. Damage to the limbic system has also led to disorders of memory, as in Korsakoff's psychosis and thiamine (vitamin B_1) deficiency found in some alcoholics.

The primary (ideotypic) sensory and motor areas of the cortex respond to the external environment. In the case of the pianist, the primary sensory cortex is not responding to (not receiving) the usual sensory feedback from his fingers when they strike the keys of the piano. The primary sensory cortex also receives sensations of light, sound, and pain from the external environment. The primary sensory and motor areas of the cortex include the primary visual cortex as well.

The unimodal association areas connect with the primary sensory and motor areas and organize sensations, such as light, into recognizable patterns (e.g., image of a face or door). The loss of blood supply caused by the stroke infarctions in the 70-year-old man had disconnected the perception of faces from previous memories of those faces. The unimodal motor association areas contain specific motor programs for complex movements, such as speaking, figure skating, piano playing, or sewing. Thus, the muscle contractions (under sensory guidance) are able to carry out learned, complex motor acts without the person having to think through each step.

The heteromodal association areas handle the cross-modal associations. They connect the unimodal and sensory association areas to the limbic system and allow communication. This allows us to assign and recall the words and names of objects, recognize and name what we touch, express our feelings, and read and write. When damage occurs to these areas, the effect can be dysnomia (impaired naming of objects, as in the 65-year-old woman), dyslexia (impaired reading), dysgraphia (impaired writing), and dyscalculia (impaired ability to calculate numbers).

The paralimbic areas form a girdle between the limbic system and the brain's heteromodal association areas described above.

75–78. The answers are 75-C, 76-E, 77-G, 78-A. *(Gatchel, 2/e, pp 233–234. Kandel, 3/e, pp 946–947. Sierles, pp 3–6, 83–91.)* George Engel (an internist and psychiatrist) proposed the biopsychosocial model in 1977. He recognized the tremendous advances being made in molecular biology and the basic biologic sciences of medicine, which he labeled the *biomedical model*. He also recognized medicine's increasingly narrow focus, so he proposed the biopsychosocial model as a broader approach, which included incorporating both the biomedical and psychosocial components as crucial to medical practice, medical education, and prevention. He proposed that all must be addressed in the consideration of the etiology, diagnosis, or treatment of each disease and each person.

Neal Miller, an American psychologist, developed (with John Dollard) a learning theory of psychotherapy that stated that fear can motivate learning. He also used a variety of behavioral techniques to study the effects of electrical and chemical stimulation of the brain (especially the hypothalamus). Perhaps most important in terms of modern behavioral medicine, he was able to prove that a variety of autonomically mediated visceral responses are subject to instrumental learning. This finding launched a whole new area of investigations that explored and demonstrated mechanisms of interaction between human behavior and human neurophysiology.

Franz Alexander (1891–1964) hypothesized that certain psychological and personality factors had a major influence on the development of certain illnesses. These illnesses were duodenal ulcer, essential hypertension, ulcerative colitis, syncope, thyrotoxicosis, rheumatic arthritis, and bronchial asthma. This represented a major step in the subsequent development of research in psychosomatic medicine. Even though the concept of a certain personality tied to a specific disease has not held up in most psychosomatic research, it has led to the identification of many psychosocial factors that interact with the disease process. Alexander also stressed the role of the therapist's personality as an important factor in psychotherapy.

Alfred Adler (1870–1937), a Viennese psychiatrist, disagreed with Freud over the dominant role of sexuality in psychopathology. He considered feelings of inferiority to be the original psychological state as a result of the infant's helpless dependency. The goal of healthy personality was to overcome feelings of inferiority. Inferiority was to be overcome by gaining power and mastery. His greatest influence was probably in the development of child guidance movements in Europe and in the United States.

Sigmund Freud (1856–1939), a Viennese psychiatrist, and founder of psychoanalysis, developed the concept of the unconscious and the technique of dream analysis. He also introduced many other concepts such as instinctual drives, death instinct, sexuality, the dominant role of psychosexual development, narcissism, catharsis, and sexually based neurotic disorders.

Harry Stack Sullivan (1892–1979) was an American psychiatrist and neopsychoanalyst. He deviated from Freud except for unconscious motivation, defense mechanisms, and dream interpretations. He considered the release of energy to be controlled by social relations and the development of personality as the result of interpersonal relations. He elaborated on the importance of self-esteem for mental health. He also insisted that the role of the therapist be one of participant-observer.

René Spitz (1897–1974) proposed that development and organization of the ego originates through the relationship between mother and child. The goal is to further the person's autonomy by progressing through a sequence of ego-organizing tasks. Social smiling, stranger anxiety, bonding with parents, and negative head-shaking are typical tasks. One of his major contributions was his study of the development of infants in a foundling home who were given good medical care, but very little contact with other human beings. These children had lower scores on developmental indices; many had anaclitic depression and very little curiosity or happiness and were prone to infections.

79–81. The answers are 79-C, 80-F, 81-A. *(Sierles, pp 55–60.)* Norepinephrine (NE) has been found to play a role in the development of depression. Most of the evidence is based on the fact that the drugs that are effective in relieving depression enhance the transmission of NE. Of the two groups of antidepressant drugs, the cyclic antidepressants block the presynaptic uptake of NE and the monoamine oxidase inhibitors block the enzymatic degradation. Furthermore, an antihypertensive drug, such as reserpine, can cause depression by disrupting the transmission of NE. This is sometimes referred to as the catecholamine hypothesis of mood disorders in which a functional deficiency of NE results in a depressed mood. While this is probably only a part of the total mood disorder equation, it is important to keep in mind that metabolic reactions can be bidirectional, and that behavior can affect the modulation of neurochemicals, as well as be affected by neurochemical reactions.

Gamma-aminobutyric acid (GABA) is an amine acid neurotransmitter that is associated with a modulating effect on anxiety. It is bound to brain receptors, and when GABA neurons fire, they dampen excitement generated in the CNS. When GABA receptors are blocked, the excitability in the brain increases, sometimes leading to seizures. When the postsynaptic receptors are bound with GABA, the chlorine channels open and the influx of chlorine negative ions hyperpolarizes the cell membrane, thus decreasing the likelihood of firing.

Acetylcholine is a neurotransmitter that is essential for memory. Persons given an anticholinergic drug that blocks acetylcholine acquire a memory deficit. When this is counteracted by another drug, memory is restored. Other studies of patients with Alzheimer's disease have confirmed the importance of acetylcholine in memory. The cholinergic hypothesis of memory has also been confirmed by pathology studies.

Behavioral Genetics

DIRECTIONS: Each question below contains five suggested responses. Select the **one best** response to each question.

82. Siblings of schizophrenics are more likely to become schizophrenic than are persons chosen randomly from the population by a factor of about

(A) 2
(B) 4
(C) 6
(D) 8
(E) 10

83. The most important (frequent) genetic cause of mental retardation is

(A) Bartholin-Patau syndrome
(B) Edwards' syndrome
(C) Down's syndrome
(D) Turner's syndrome
(E) Klinefelter's syndrome

84. Which of the following studies is most effective in estimating the genetic risk of an alcoholic offspring's becoming an alcoholic if adopted or raised by a nonalcoholic family?

(A) Family studies
(B) Studies of twins reared together
(C) Adopted twin studies
(D) Nontwin adoption studies
(E) Pedigree and linkage studies

85. A person with Klinefelter's syndrome has the genotype

(A) XY
(B) YY
(C) XXY
(D) XYY
(E) XXX

86. Heredity accounts for approximately what percentage of total variation in IQ scores within a family?

(A) 5 percent
(B) 25 percent
(C) 50 percent
(D) 75 percent
(E) 100 percent

87. From studies of twins reared together and reared apart, which of the following characteristics has been confirmed as having the highest heritability?

(A) Aggressiveness
(B) Extroversion
(C) Empathy
(D) Stress reaction
(E) Neuroticism

88. The complex of severe psychologic disorders known as schizophrenia has a demonstrable basis that is characterized as

(A) environmentally determined
(B) polygenic
(C) a chromosomal aberration
(D) a simple recessive trait
(E) an inborn error of metabolism

89. A disorder resulting from a single gene defect that may produce severe mental problems is

(A) manic-depressive psychosis
(B) dyslexia
(C) phenylketonuria
(D) Porter's syndrome
(E) Down's syndrome

DIRECTIONS: Each numbered question or incomplete statement below is NEGATIVELY phrased. Select the **one best** lettered response.

90. The prominence of genetic factors in alcoholism is illustrated by all the following findings EXCEPT that

(A) close relatives of alcoholics have a fourfold increased risk

(B) an alcoholic's children who are given up for adoption at birth are at fourfold increased risk

(C) the risk for the identical twin of an alcoholic is much higher than for a fraternal twin

(D) close relatives of alcoholics are significantly more vulnerable for other psychiatric illnesses

(E) children of an alcoholic become less intoxicated at a given alcohol level than do controls

91. Genetic factors are most likely to predispose a person to alcoholism by increasing any of the following EXCEPT

(A) positive reinforcement of alcohol consumption

(B) functional tolerance of alcohol

(C) level of alcohol dependence

(D) rate of alcohol metabolism

(E) level of acetylaldehyde

92. Factors that influence a person's gender identity include all the following EXCEPT

(A) chromosomal configuration (XX or XY)

(B) gender assigned at birth

(C) internal reproductive structures

(D) role model of parent

(E) response of parent to child's assigned gender

93. Ethology is characterized by all the following concepts EXCEPT

(A) behavior is best studied under controlled conditions

(B) behavior is best studied comparatively

(C) behavior is the result of interaction between genetic endowment and environment

(D) innate behavior is triggered by a sign stimulus or releaser

(E) previous learning is unnecessary for the successful expression of a fixed action pattern

94. Of the following illnesses or syndromes, which is LEAST related to genetic factors?

(A) Schizophrenia

(B) Panic disorder

(C) Bipolar disorder

(D) Alcoholism

(E) Antisocial personality

95. Ethology has made major contributions to understanding human behavior through all the following concepts EXCEPT

(A) fixed action pattern
(B) critical period
(C) imprinting
(D) ethnic bonds
(E) sign stimulus

96. Emotional expressions involving a stereotyped sequence of fixed action patterns include all the following EXCEPT

(A) smiling
(B) brow flash response
(C) startle response
(D) apprehension
(E) joy

97. Which of the following is LEAST likely to be considered an ontogenetic stage of synaptic development and modification?

(A) Synapse formation under genetic and developmental control
(B) Maintenance of newly developed synapses occurring during critical periods
(C) Regulation of transient and long-term effectiveness of synapses
(D) Integration of cellular structure for human mentation
(E) Alteration of preexisting pathways and development of new patterns

98. Human behavioral patterns that have the potential of containing major innate (i.e., genetic, or not learned) components include all the following EXCEPT

(A) intelligence
(B) brow flash response
(C) facial expressions of anger, fear, disgust, and joy
(D) smiling
(E) handshake greeting

DIRECTIONS: The group of questions below consists of lettered headings followed by a set of numbered items. For each numbered item select the **one** lettered heading with which it is **most** closely associated. Each lettered heading may be used **once, more than once, or not at all.**

Questions 99–101

For each later condition or behavior listed below, select the most closely associated early predictor.

(A) Birth weight
(B) Handedness
(C) Temperament
(D) Age of mother at birth
(E) Intelligence
(F) Malnutrition
(G) Aggressiveness
(H) Assertiveness

99. School performance

100. Need for psychiatric care

101. Adolescent and young adult violence

Behavioral Genetics
Answers

82. The answer is D. *(Plomin, 2/e, pp 303–307.)* The risk of schizophrenia in the general population is about 1 percent. Studies of the risks for relatives of schizophrenics reveal that schizophrenia runs in families. Siblings of schizophrenics are approximately eight times more likely to become schizophrenic than are persons chosen randomly from the population; this rate almost doubles when those siblings have an affected parent as well as an affected sibling. The risk is no greater when the mother is schizophrenic than when the father is schizophrenic. If both parents are schizophrenic, the risk becomes four times as great as when only one parent is schizophrenic. Grandchildren of schizophrenics have about twice the risk as the general population since grandchildren share about one-fourth of the grandparent's segregating genes; great-grandchildren (sharing about one-eighth of the genes) have a slightly more than average chance of becoming schizophrenic.

83. The answer is C. *(Plomin, 2/e, pp 130–136.)* Almost all chromosomal abnormalities influence general cognitive ability and growth. Down's syndrome is the most frequent genetic cause of mental retardation. It often bears a strong relationship to maternal age. Persons with Down's syndrome have 47 chromosomes instead of the normal 46. The syndrome was originally named trisomy 21 because, at the time, the trisomy was thought to involve the next to the smallest autosome (number 21 by the Denver system of enumeration). It is now known that the smallest autosome is the one in triplicate. Even though Down's syndrome should really be called trisomy 22, the error is so firmly entrenched in the literature that it is still referred to as involving chromosome 21. Turner's syndrome (XO) occurs in females with the absence of one of the two X chromosomes. Although most sufferers have a normal IQ, Turner's syndrome nearly always involves sterility, with some limited secondary sexual development. Persons with Klinefelter's syndrome (XXY) are phenotypic males with an extra X chromosome. About 1 percent of males institutionalized for retardation have Klinefelter's syndrome. Bartholin-Patau syndrome (trisomy 13) and Edwards' syndrome (trisomy 18) are caused by trisomy of chromosomes 13 and 18, respectively. Sufferers are characterized as severely retarded, and most die in the first few months of life.

84. The answer is D. *(Sierles, pp 64–65.)* A nontwin adoption study can be most helpful in determining the effect of being raised by a nonalcoholic family on the offspring of an alcoholic parent. The genetic effect of having an alcoholic biologic parent can be determined by longitudinally observing the rate of alcoholism in the offspring of alcoholic parents who were adopted by (raised by) nonalcoholic families and comparing it with the rate of alcoholism in adopted children of nonalcoholic biologic parents. A higher rate of alcoholism will occur in the adopted children of alcoholic parents, but it will be less than that of those raised by an alcoholic parent. A similar strategy can determine the effect of having a biologic parent who is mentally ill, but of being raised by a parent who is not mentally ill. A cross-fostering variation of nontwin adoption studies can also determine the effect of being reared by a mentally ill parent.

85. The answer is C. *(Plomin, 2/e, pp 141–143.)* Persons with Klinefelter's syndrome, a genetic disorder of men, exhibit a variety of male morphological and behavioral characteristics. This phenomenon is attributed to the extra X (male) chromosome in such a person's genotype (XXY). These persons represent nearly 1 percent of males institutionalized for retardation, epilepsy, or mental illness; the incidence in the general population is 2 per 1000 newborn males. They generally have abnormally small testes, low levels of male hormone (testosterone), and sterility. In spite of a high incidence of mental retardation, about 75 percent have IQs within the normal range.

86. The answer is C. *(Plomin, 2/e, pp 297–303.)* Studies of several decades ago calculated that heritability accounted for about 70 to 75 percent of the total variation in IQ scores within a family. More recent studies involving much larger samples show that the individual differences in general cognitive ability within families are actually closer to 50 percent. Inheritance is still a major factor in the development of individual differences in IQ, since no specific environmental influence has been found to account for even as much as 10 percent of the variance in IQ scores within families.

87. The answer is A. *(Sierles, pp 66–68.)* Aggressivenesss—the readiness to argue or fight or even to be vindictive—has been shown by studies of monozygotic (MZ) and dizygotic (DZ) twins reared together and apart to have a high heritability. Extroversion, empathy, and neuroticism have been found to have a high heritability in twins reared together, but not in twins reared apart. Similarly, stress reaction (feeling vulnerable or given to worry) has been found to have a high heritability whether twins are reared together or apart, but not as high as aggressiveness. Many traits of MZ and DZ twins have been found to have a high heritability of 39 to 58 percent, whether the twins were reared together or apart.

88. The answer is B. *(Plomin, 2/e, pp 303–307.)* Complex behavioral traits such as schizophrenia, which may vary widely in nature from person to person, are considered to involve anomalies at more than one gene locus. The science of behavior genetics deals with the quantitative analysis of these polygenic traits. The results of a great variety of investigations now favor the view that schizophrenia is a genetically determined disorder, but it also may be substantially affected by environmental influences.

89. The answer is C. *(Plomin, 2/e, pp 8–9, 66–67.)* Phenylketonuria (PKU) results from the inheritance of a double recessive gene. Affected persons suffer an inability to metabolize phenylalanine, a common amino acid in food. If the condition is undetected in time for treatment with special diets, serious mental deficiency results, presumably as a consequence of the toxic effect of abnormal blood levels of phenylpyruvic acid on the developing brain. About 1 percent of institutionalized retarded persons are retarded because of PKU. Most persons with PKU do not become mentally retarded if they are given a diet low in phenylalanine during the developing years. Early identification of affected infants combined with replacement of milk with galactose-free substances has been quite successful in reducing the subsequent mental retardation. PKU is a good example of genes affecting behavior in the same way genes affect phenotypes. Its treatment also provides an example of an environmental intervention successfully bypassing a genetic problem.

90. The answer is D. *(Isselbacher, 13/e, p 2423.)* Family, twin, and adoption studies support the importance of genetic factors in alcoholism. Close relatives of alcoholics have a fourfold increased risk, which is still true even if the children of alcoholics are given up for adoption at birth without the alcohol problems of their parents being known. The fourfold increased risk of close relatives for alcoholism does not make them significantly more vulnerable for other psychiatric illnesses. Twin research has shown that the risk for the identical twin of an alcoholic is much higher than for a fraternal twin. Other studies suggest that the children of an alcoholic become less intoxicated at the same blood alcohol level than do controls. This occurs even before alcoholism develops.

91. The answer is E. *(Linden, pp 22–24.)* Studies have demonstrated that animals can be selectively bred for their preference for and consumption of alcohol and for their susceptibility to the effects of alcohol upon the central nervous system. Individual differences also occur in the amount of acquired functional tolerance and positive reinforcement. The rate of metabolism is more concordant in monozygotic twins than in dizygotic twins. Alcohol dehydrogenase (ADH) metabolizes alcohol and results in an increased level of toxic acetylaldehyde. This acts to suppress alcohol consumption, presumably through aversion control. Studies have also shown that some aspects of dependence are heritable, especially severity of dependence and craving for alcohol.

92. The answer is B. *(Schuster, 3/e, p 301.)* Seven significant variables potentially influence one's gender identity. They are (1) chromosomal configuration (XX or XY), (2) gonad endowment (ovaries or testes), (3) internal reproductive structures (uterus or prostate), (4) external genitalia (vagina or penis), (5) hormonal balance (estrogen or androgen), (6) gender assigned at birth, and (7) response of the parents to the child's assigned gender. The role model of either parent is an important influence on a person's gender behavior but not on gender identity, which occurs earlier than the learning of gender behavior.

93. The answer is A. *(Kandel, 3/e, pp 987–995.)* Ethology was developed by Konrad Lorenz and Nicholaas Tinbergen during the period from 1920 to 1950 by conducting comparative studies of unlearned behavior with special emphasis on its mechanisms, ontogeny, and evolution. They emphasized the observation of behavior under natural conditions and recognized that all behavior is the result of the interaction between the animal's genetic endowment and the animal's internal and external environment. Innate behavior is a relatively complex sequence of responses, called a *fixed action pattern*, which is triggered by a sign stimulus or releaser. Thus behavior patterns (e.g., mating) in lower animals can be activated by a specific stimulus (e.g., the male stickleback fish develops a bright red abdomen [the sign stimulus] that triggers mating behavior [fixed action patterns] of the female). A fixed action pattern, somewhat like a reflex, does not require previous learning for its expression.

94. The answer is B. *(Sierles, p 66.)* Using family heritance, twin, and adoption studies, schizophrenia, bipolar disorder, alcoholism, and antisocial personality have all been demonstrated to have genetic factors. On the other hand, panic disorder has been shown to have a familial factor but has not been demonstrated to be strongly genetic by monozygotic and dizygotic twin and adoption studies. Other illnesses or syndromes with strong genetic components are unipolar disorder, depression, anorexia nervosa, obsessive-compulsive disorders, and some anxiety disorders.

95. The answer is D. *(Kandel, 3/e, pp 987–991.)* Ethology in psychology and biology has made a number of conceptual contributions to understanding human behavior through the comparative study of animal behavior in relation to natural habitat. Ethologists have found evidence to suggest that some aspects of human behavior may be a function of species membership in the form of predispositions to learn and respond in certain ways rather than the fixed sequences of motor activity found in lower animals. The fixed action pattern is a genetically established sequence of motor activity that is triggered by a sign stimulus that is sufficient to release the fixed action pattern of behavior. These links between sign stimulus and fixed action pattern are weaker and more variable in humans because of the overriding effects of experience and learning. However, certain predispositions to respond to certain stimuli in certain ways are presently being explored. Imprinting is the tendency of very young animals to become fixed on and follow a member of their own species (usually their mother, but another animal or even an object can be substituted). The period of development when there is maximum receptivity to these crucial cues is known as the critical period. Bond formation between infants and adults does occur in both humans and lower animals, but ethnic bonds appear to be almost totally learned rather than biologically established.

96. The answer is D. *(Kandel, 3/e, pp 990–995.)* Humans have a number of simple behaviors that resemble the fixed action patterns of lower animals. Such emotional expressions as the startle response and smiling are stereotyped sequences of movements. In human infants smiling appears to be under the control of a specific sign stimulus. Studies show that the smiling response is not triggered by the face as a whole, but rather by certain specific features. For example, the eyes are of particular importance as a sign stimulus, and as the child matures, other features of the face become important. The brow flash response (rapid raising and dropping of eyebrows) is a stereotyped response present in widely different cultures and is used as part of a greeting response. A complex set of human behaviors that is universal in emotional expression across cultures and that involves a stereotyped sequence of fixed action patterns includes the facial expressions of anger, fear, disgust, and joy. As an example, babies who are born blind can have emotional facial expressions that appear normal. While apprehension may include some of the responses also found in fear, it does not include as many as found in fear, nor are the responses as severe.

97. The answer is D. *(Kandel, 3/e, pp 945–957.)* In general, there are at least three ontogenetic stages of synaptic modification. The first is the stage of synapse formation, which occurs under genetic and developmental control. The next stage is that of maintaining and "fine tuning" of the newly developed synapses during early critical periods of development. This requires an appropriate pattern of environmental stimulation. The third stage is the regulation of the transient and long-term effectiveness of the synapses, which takes place throughout life as one initiates and accumulates day-to-day behavioral experience. An overall stage involving environmental and learning factors brings out the latent and potential capabilities for all behaviors by altering the effectiveness of preexisting neural pathways and effecting the expression of new patterns of behavior.

98. The answer is E. *(Kandel, 3/e, pp 993–995.)* Even though most research on innate behavior has been done on nonmammalian species, nonhuman primates also exhibit innate behavior with innate releasing mechanisms. Some studies with humans demonstrated innate (i.e., genetic, or not learned) determinants of human behavior (e.g., hormonal determinants of gender identity). Since genes control so much of the formation and organization of the basic components of all behavior, including human behavior, behavior must to some extent be under genetic control. Inherited factors nearly always depend on the interaction of genetic and environmental factors in order to be expressed. Some severe mental illnesses, such as schizophrenia, Down's syndrome, and bipolar depression, have known hereditary factors. Intelligence also has a strong genetic component. Certain human behaviors are universal across cultures — for example, deep tendon reflexes, the eyeblink, and startle reflexes. There are also common drives and needs — for example, hunger, thirst, and sex, and probably the need for social contact and a number of sensory experiences. Certain emotional expressions and facial motor patterns are also universal — for example, facial expressions of anger, fear, disgust, and joy. Infant smiling is a stereotyped behavior that appears to be controlled by a specific sign stimulus, not always in response to another smiling human face. The brow flash response is also stereotyped and consists of a rapid raising and dropping of the eyebrows as a part of the greeting response between persons who know each other, while a handshake is a learned cultural behavior.

99–101. The answers are 99–E, 100–C, 101–G. *(Sierles, pp 66–71, 128–131, 358–363.)* Childhood behaviors or conditions often predict later behaviors. Childhood intelligence tends to predict later school performance. Since there is a high heritability of IQ (50 to 70 percent) and school performance depends heavily on specific cognitive abilities such as verbal ability, spatial ability, learning, and retention, early demonstration of these attributes will predict higher school performance in the future.

Temperaments expressed during childhood are predictive of adult temperaments, and persons with difficult temperaments are more apt to require later psychiatric care. The measurement of temperament has nine components: activity level, rhythmicity (the regularity of body functions, such as sleep and eating), tendency to approach or withdraw from new persons or situations, adaptability, response to stimulation, intensity, quality of mood (whether the subject is pleased, friendly, crying, unfriendly), distractibility, and attention span. For example, the difficult child (about 10 percent) will demonstrate intense reactions, show irregularity of functions, tend to withdraw, and adapt poorly. Even though temperament has a heritable component, the environment and especially interpersonal relationships with parents and their expectations can modify and "harness" a difficult temperament.

Aggression in childhood can predict future expressions of aggression and violence in adolescence and adulthood. This higher expectancy of continued aggression and violence is in part related to heritability confirmed by studies of twins whether reared together or apart. Other studies have also confirmed that family environment has a strong influence on the transition of aggression and antisocial behavior into violence. For example, the risk of antisocial and violent behavior in adulthood is increased by low social status, low educational attainment, lax or inconsistent or severe discipline, instability of early home environment, and being reared by a violent or criminal parent. The triad of male, young, and poor is overrepresented in the perpetrators of violence and in the victims of violence. The principle that past behavior tends to predict future behavior still holds.

Individual Behavior and Personality

DIRECTIONS: Each question below contains four or five suggested responses. Select the **one best** response to each question.

102. The psychosocial factor most prominent in a person who is engaging in substance abuse is

(A) delusions of grandeur
(B) depressed mood
(C) rationalization
(D) denial
(E) antisocial behavior

103. Which of the following negative emotional states or conditions most commonly precedes relapse in the treatment of addictive behaviors?

(A) Stress
(B) Depression
(C) Anxiety
(D) Anger
(E) Frustration

104. Although there is no uniform asthmatic personality type, the most frequent psychological characteristic of boys with bronchial asthma is

(A) hostility
(B) general anxiety
(C) frustrated oral needs
(D) dependency
(E) latent homosexuality

105. According to psychoanalytic theory, which of the following statements about the development of the superego is true?

(A) It is present at birth
(B) It begins to develop during the first 2 years of life
(C) It begins to develop during the fifth or sixth year of life
(D) It begins to develop during puberty
(E) It begins to develop in late adolescence

106. Freud maintained that neuroses were primarily a result of

(A) overly severe toilet training
(B) inappropriate identification
(C) primary processes
(D) inadequate superego development
(E) sexual disturbances

107. Freud maintained that interruptions in the flow of free association were indicative of which of the following?

(A) Reaction formation
(B) Resistance
(C) Repression
(D) Parapraxis
(E) The pleasure principle

108. The most common mental disorder in the U.S. population is

(A) phobic disorder
(B) anxiety disorder
(C) schizophrenia
(D) mood disorder
(E) obsessive-compulsive disorder

109. A 30-year-old man with recently developed AIDS is referred to you as a primary care physician. What is apt to be the most prominent psychosocial factor or reaction that you can expect and perhaps help prevent?

(A) Loss of independence
(B) Fear of losing confidentiality
(C) Guilt
(D) Depressed mood
(E) Suicidal thoughts

110. In traditional psychoanalysis, transference is the process wherein

(A) psychic energy, or libido, is transferred from the id to the ego and superego
(B) a patient invests the analyst with attitudes and feelings derived from vital earlier associations
(C) certain psychological symptoms seemingly defer to new symptoms that frequently are more accessible to analysis
(D) early object choices are gradually decathected
(E) latent dream content is transformed into manifest content

111. The thematic apperception test (TAT) would be most useful for which of the following purposes?

(A) As an aid in differential diagnosis
(B) In prediction of suitability for psychotherapy
(C) In assessment of suicidal risk
(D) In assessment of intellectual level
(E) In assessment of motivational variables

112. In the assessment of personality, the normative and objective method refers to

(A) the use of "inkblot" techniques
(B) sophisticated techniques for measuring the accuracy of a person's perception of reality
(C) predictions of behavior on the basis of intensive interviewing
(D) predictions of behavior on the basis of data from personality tests
(E) a way of evaluating personality rather than of simply assessing how a person behaves

113. Among combat veterans, the greatest risk for posttraumatic stress disorder is among those who

(A) were violent prior to service
(B) have a prior history of depression
(C) have coexisting sociopathy
(D) participated in noncombatant violence
(E) have a history of substance abuse

114. In Freudian theory, patients suffering from obsessive-compulsive neurosis customarily display which of the following behavior patterns?

(A) Explosive outbursts of temper
(B) Isolation, undoing, and reaction formation
(C) Conversion of psychological conflicts to somatic symptoms
(D) Willingness to engage in antisocial activities and in deviant sexual activity
(E) None of the above

115. A person with which of the following mental disorders is most apt to seek medical help?

(A) Major depressive disorder
(B) Bipolar depressive disorder
(C) Dysthymic disorder
(D) Panic disorder
(E) Obsessive-compulsive disorder

116. According to Freud, the superego contains the

(A) conscience
(B) pleasure principle
(C) ego instincts
(D) reality principle
(E) internalized ego

117. Which of the following type A, or coronary-prone, behavioral factors appears to be the most important?

(A) Hostility
(B) Competitiveness
(C) Time urgency
(D) Explosive speech
(E) Hyperactivity

118. Which of the following defense mechanisms is most frequently observed on the medical and surgical wards?

(A) Rationalization
(B) Projection
(C) Displacement
(D) Sublimation
(E) Denial

119. Patients who have somatization disorder are diagnosed on the basis of their

(A) having unexplained symptoms that persist after treatment
(B) experiencing symptoms in multiple organ systems
(C) having a history of past and present illnesses that have not responded to self-treatment
(D) having a specific number of medically unexplained symptoms
(E) demonstrating positive test results for several chronic illnesses at the same time

120. The most frequent psychiatric disorder of postpartum women is

(A) an episode of mild schizophrenia
(B) an episode of mania
(C) postpartum blues
(D) major depression
(E) postpartum psychosis

121. The importance of unconscious determinants was most strongly emphasized by which one of the following personality theorists?

(A) B. F. Skinner
(B) Carl Jung
(C) Kurt Lewin
(D) Henry Murray
(E) Margaret Mead

122. Which of the following methods of assessment would be most useful in the detection of brain damage?

(A) Thematic apperception test
(B) Bender-Gestalt test
(C) California personality inventory
(D) Minnesota multiphasic personality inventory (MMPI)
(E) Millon behavioral health inventory (MBHI)

123. The highest compliance with medication treatment is found in which of the following illnesses?

(A) Diabetes
(B) Cancer
(C) Hypertension
(D) Coronary heart disease
(E) Glaucoma

124. Contrary to coping mechanisms, defense mechanisms

(A) confront a problem directly and continue to generate possible solutions
(B) get help when one is unable to handle the problem
(C) work to remove awareness of the conflict
(D) consciously drop certain habits or form new ones
(E) gather information

DIRECTIONS: Each numbered question or incomplete statement below is NEGATIVELY phrased. Select the **one best** lettered response.

125. Patients with a strong sense of an external locus of control of health will be more apt to respond to inpatient treatment in all the following ways EXCEPT

(A) they delegate control of their health to their doctor or significant other
(B) they can be relied on to follow treatment orders when they are discharged for outpatient follow-up
(C) they respond well and more comfortably to inpatient care
(D) they prefer to make as few decisions about their care as possible
(E) they prefer to make few decisions about their own health care

126. Patients with a strong perception of an internal locus of control regarding health are more apt to respond to their physicians and to outpatient treatment in all the following ways EXCEPT

(A) they willingly accept the authority of their own physician regarding inpatient treatment
(B) they make personal adjustments in the diet prescribed by their own physician
(C) they make independent decisions on drug dosages prescribed by their physician
(D) they consider themselves and the physician to be a team

127. Illness tends to activate all the following EXCEPT

(A) dependence on other people
(B) recall of relationships of early childhood
(C) sense of vulnerability
(D) sense of control
(E) helplessness

128. True statements about personality traits and aging include all the following EXCEPT

(A) a person's personality traits after age 30 tend to be less variable
(B) the personalities of adolescents show lower levels of stability than those of adults
(C) most people redefine and make alterations in their personalities during the period of midlife crisis
(D) the neuroticism trait in personality has a high correlation with lower levels of stability
(E) personality traits are relatively stable over one's life span

129. Hypochondriacal patients tend to exhibit each of the following EXCEPT

(A) quick improvement with treatment
(B) dependent personalities
(C) depression
(D) anxiety
(E) chronic reaction to stress as a "way of life"

130. The obese person is LEAST responsive to which of the following cues?

(A) Gastric contraction
(B) Taste
(C) Smell
(D) Attractiveness of food
(E) Abundance of food

131. Which of the following will be LEAST constant from middle to old age?

(A) Emotional stability
(B) Sociability
(C) Assertiveness
(D) Selfishness
(E) Wisdom

132. In the health belief model, the patient's compliance is LEAST affected by the

(A) patient's analysis of costs and benefits
(B) patient's perception of severity of the illness
(C) patient's readiness to act
(D) cue to action
(E) objective characteristics of the illness

133. In Carl Rogers's personality theory, the LEAST important component of a psychotherapeutic process involves

(A) a therapist's empathy
(B) a therapist's unconditional positive regard
(C) interpretation of unconscious wishes and feelings
(D) reflection of a client's feelings
(E) clarification of conflictive feelings and attitudes

134. All the following are examples of projective tests EXCEPT

(A) thematic apperception test (TAT)
(B) draw-a-person test
(C) sentence completion test
(D) Rorschach test
(E) Minnesota multiphasic personality inventory (MMPI)

135. Frequent behavioral manifestations that may be helpful in identifying a girl who has been sexually abused include all the following EXCEPT

(A) simulation of sex acts with dolls
(B) increase of hugging and body touching
(C) inclusion of genitalia in drawings
(D) verbal references to molestation
(E) sleep or phobia disorders

136. All the following statements about schizophrenia are true EXCEPT that

(A) twin, family, and adoption studies have demonstrated that schizophrenia has a significant genetic basis

(B) higher socioeconomic status correlates positively with the incidence of schizophrenia

(C) auditory hallucinations are frequently present

(D) chlorpromazine is an effective form of treatment

(E) communication conflicts in families of schizophrenics play an etiologic role

137. All the following are tenets of psychoanalytic theory EXCEPT that

(A) all mental events and attitudes have unconscious antecedent causes

(B) a significant portion of the contents of the mind is unconscious

(C) normal and pathologic mental functioning are qualitatively different

(D) people strive to maximize pleasure and minimize tension

(E) early experience is important in the formation of individual personality

138. All the following statements about anxiety are true EXCEPT that

(A) intense, manifest anxiety reactions usually involve cardiovascular, respiratory, and gastrointestinal changes

(B) anxiety as subjectively experienced bears no consistent relationship to physiologic responses commonly associated with it

(C) anticipation of a stressful event usually reduces the actual level of anxiety the event evokes

(D) performance levels rise and fall with anxiety levels in a linear fashion

(E) avoidance behavior is reinforced when it reduces an anxiety state

DIRECTIONS: Each group of questions below consists of lettered headings followed by a set of numbered items. For each numbered item select the **one** lettered heading with which it is **most** closely associated. Each lettered heading may be used **once, more than once, or not at all.**

Questions 139–142

For each of the descriptions below, select the psychological test with which it is most closely associated

(A) Halstead-Reitan battery (HRB)
(B) Wechsler adult intelligence scale (WAIS)
(C) Minnesota multiphasic personality inventory (MMPI)
(D) Thematic apperception test (TAT)
(E) Bender-Gestalt test

139. Assesses visual motor coordination

140. Provides scores on ten standardized clinical scales so as to separate medical or psychiatric patients from normal controls

141. Determines the location and effects of specific brain lesions

142. Consists of six verbal subtests and five performance subtests

Questions 143–145

For each pairing of unconscious attitude and conscious attitude that "conceals" it, choose the defense mechanism to which it most closely corresponds.

(A) Reaction formation
(B) Undoing
(C) Denial
(D) Projection
(E) Isolation

143. I hate him (unconscious); I love him (conscious)

144. I hate him (unconscious); he hates me (conscious)

145. I hate him (unconscious); I don't hate him (conscious)

Questions 146–149

For each combination of sibling relatedness and rearing, select the IQ coefficient with which it is most closely associated.

(A) 0.86
(B) 0.72
(C) 0.60
(D) 0.47
(E) 0.24

146. Fraternal twins reared together

147. Identical twins reared together

148. Identical twins reared apart

149. Siblings reared together

Questions 150–152

For each concept relating to stress, select the investigator or team of investigators with whom it is most closely associated.

(A) Hans Selye
(B) Walter Cannon
(C) Hippocrates
(D) John Mason and Marianne Frankenhauser
(E) Richard Lazarus

150. Emotional and physiologic response to danger

151. General adaptation syndrome

152. Psychological appraisal of a potentially stressful event or stimulus followed by coping strategies and/or reappraisal

Questions 153–155

Match each of the statements linking heart disease to stress and type A behavior with the correct researcher or team of researchers.

(A) Karen Mathews
(B) Richard Rosenman and Milton Friedman
(C) D. R. Ragland and R. J. Brand
(D) David Glass
(E) David Jenkins

153. Developed a self-report survey of activity to assess type A behavior

154. Emphasized type A pattern as a coping style used to establish and maintain control over stressful situations

155. Developed a measure of type A behavior in children and adolescents

Questions 156–159

For each patient described, select the most appropriate personality disorder.

(A) Schizoid

(B) Schizotypal

(C) Paranoid

(D) Histrionic

(E) Antisocial

(F) Avoidant

(G) Dependent

(H) Passive-aggressive

(I) Borderline

(J) Obsessive-compulsive

(K) Narcissistic

156. A 30-year-old warehouse clerk helps himself to selected items because he feels that the management is overcharging and robbing the customers

157. A 40-year-old unemployed salesman has superficial charm but is easily irritated; he lost his job because he was intentionally abusive to the boss's dog

158. An 18-year-old female student was found perched atop the belltower balcony of her high school; she told the fire chief that she hated her parents and that she felt empty and alone

159. A 35-year-old bookkeeper in a construction firm has become increasingly frustrated and unhappy with his job over the past 10 years and with the people for whom he has been working, and he complains constantly to his few friends; he finds himself dawdling, procrastinating, forgetting, and arriving late for work, but as his mistakes at work increase, he feels less guilt about them

Individual Behavior and Personality

Answers

102. The answer is D. *(Sierles, pp 295–296.)* Even though there is no single personality type associated with substance abuse, denial is the major psychosocial factor in these persons. Denial can also complicate the treatment, even though the substance abuser may admit to the addiction. Substance abusers do frequently display delusions of grandeur, are often in a depressed mood, frequently display antisocial behavior, and often rationalize their behavior or situation, but denying the seriousness of their drinking or drug problem and its effect on their life or loved ones is the most common psychosocial factor seen. Denial is a form of self-deception that permeates their psychological and social behavior. A physician must be constantly aware of the influence of denial on the patient's self-reported history and the effect of denial on prognosis.

103. The answer is C. *(Linden, pp 292–294.)* Negative emotional states of anxiety, anger, frustration, depression, and stress are related to relapse in the treatment of addictive behaviors involved in such disorders as alcoholism, smoking, obesity, and drug addiction. Most patients (about 70 percent) have negative affects preceding the relapse. The most common negative affect or mood state is anxiety, followed by anger or frustration, and depression. Furthermore, patients are at increased risk for relapse if they smoke, drink, eat, and so on in an attempt to reduce negative affect.

104. The answer is D. *(Kaplan, 7/e, p 759.)* Clinical research has determined that the historical formulation of the so-called asthmatic personality is not valid. Psychological factors are important, however, and it has been determined that about one-half of the patients with asthma have strong unconscious wishes for protection centering on persons on whom they are dependent. Threat of loss or separation from the mother can produce attacks of bronchial asthma in some persons, whereas in others the wish for protection produces an intense conflict, so that separation can actually produce a remission from an attack. Asthmatic boys, rather than girls, tend to be more dependent on their mothers, whereas asthmatic girls tend to be more dependent on their fathers. Although girls may try to be self-sufficient, they are frequently chronically depressed. Boys are also apt to be passively dependent, timid, and immature. Both, however, appear to be dominated by a fear of losing parental support. Studies have found that about 50 percent of all asthmatic attacks, regardless of a patient's age at the time of occurrence, are initiated or precipitated by actual or anticipated separation from or loss of the person on whom he or she is dependent.

105. The answer is C. *(Kaplan, 7/e, pp 247–248.)* Freud maintained that the superego begins to develop around the age of 5 or 6 as part of the resolution of the Oedipus complex. At the end of the phallic stage of psychosexual development (which lasts from around $2\frac{1}{2}$ to 6 years of age), children must abandon the sexual and aggressive impulses that were directed toward their parents in order to avoid the parents' strong disapproval. In abandoning these impulses, children identify with their parents. Part of this identification involves the internalization of parental standards of morality; this internalization marks the beginning of the superego.

106. The answer is E. *(Lerner, Encyclopedia, pp 375–377.)* Although Freud modified many aspects of his theory of neuroses, he never wavered in his conviction that sexual disturbances were the most important causal factor in neurotic development. One of the first to recognize the existence of sexual feelings and curiosity in children, Freud maintained that in the course of socialization some of a child's sexual feelings become repressed. Occasionally, the act of repression reaches extreme proportions, consuming enormous amounts of psychic energy. Freud believed that under stress, this repression often would fail, allowing the sexual impulses, partially freed, to appear in the form of neurotic symptoms.

107. The answer is B. *(Lerner, Psychology, pp 511–513.)* One of the most important techniques in psychoanalysis is free association, in which a patient is encouraged to say whatever comes to mind, however absurd or objectionable it might seem. This can be a difficult undertaking. Frequently, the flow of associations is interrupted and a patient's train of thought is blocked or lost because of resistance, which is a defensive maneuver that prevents repressed material from emerging into consciousness.

108. The answer is B. *(Sierles, pp 255–266.)* Anxiety disorders are the most common mental disorders in the U.S.; 4 to 14 percent of general medical patients suffer from anxiety states. Patients with anxiety disorders are more apt to seek help from general physicians or to use the emergency room than are patients with other psychiatric disorders. Mood disorders are the second most common mental disorders in the U.S.; they afflict 5 percent at any point in time, with a 1-year prevalence of 9.5 percent for all mood disorders. Prevalence of mood disorders among patients seeking help in a primary care outpatient setting range from 4.8 to 8.6 percent for major depressive disorder, and 2.1 to 8.7 percent for dysthymic disorder. That adds up to 10.2 to 21 percent of primary care outpatients who suffer from clinically significant mood disorders. They are also high users of nonpsychiatric medical and primary care and of emergency services. Anxiety disorders and mood disorders should be a part of the differential diagnosis when a patient seeks help for depressive symptoms.

109. The answer is D. *(Sierles, pp 9–11.)* A depressed mood and depressive illnesses are the most common psychosocial reactions of persons with AIDS. A depressive illness can be secondary to a viral infection of the brain and nervous system or a side effect of drugs used to treat AIDS, or it can arise from preexisting mood disorders. Depressed mood and depressive illnesses can also occur from psychosocial stress generated from such factors as reception of a fatal diagnosis, loss of confidentiality, stigma of having AIDS, rejection by friends and family, loss of independence, loss of bowel and bladder control, or loss of occupational competence. Adaptation is a psychosocial factor that affects depression, especially in terms of what the illness means to the patient — e.g., the illness as a challenge, an enemy, a punishment, a weakness, a strategy for life, an irreparable loss or injury, an incentive to change behavior, or a threat to coping capacities. Some of the behaviors that can be observed in depressed moods and illnesses include a sad, apathetic, or anxious mood, loss of self-esteem, guilt, hopeless or helpless feelings, insomnia, loss of appetite, and suicidal thoughts.

110. The answer is B. *(Kaplan, 7/e, pp 826–827.)* In traditional psychoanalytic treatment, analysts purposely reveal very little about themselves to their patients. That is intended to help promote transference — to create an ambiance that facilitates a patient's ability to transfer his or her past emotional attachments to the psychoanalyst. The analyst becomes a substitute for the parental figure. In positive transference, the patient becomes attached to the analyst in order to obtain love and emotional satisfaction, whereas in negative transference the analyst is seen as an unfair, unloving, and rejecting parental figure. Interpretations of transference may help the patient see the positive or negative feelings as a reflection of previous emotional entanglements.

111. The answer is E. *(Kaplan, 7/e, p 229.)* The thematic apperception test (TAT), which consists of a series of 30 ambiguous pictures about which subjects are asked to construct a story, is most useful in assessing motivational variables. It provides a case-study exploration of a person's personality. Although it also has been employed to assess variables such as intellectual level, other tests are more suitable for such purposes (e.g., IQ tests). The TAT is not particularly helpful in differential diagnosis.

112. The answer is D. *(Kaplan, 7/e, pp 223–227.)* Normative and objective methods involve statistical prediction based on quantified data. Applied to the assessment of personality, such methods are independent of any particular theory of personality, relying on the use of a mathematical relationship between relevant test scores and a particular behavioral outcome that is to be predicted. The 1950s and 1960s witnessed a controversy over the relative merits of personality assessment and prediction on the basis of clinical interviewing techniques versus those of actuarial and statistical data. Today, researchers and clinicians usually view these procedures as complementary, and both methods currently are employed for different types of research or personality assessment.

113. The answer is D. *(Sierles, pp 264–266.)* Posttraumatic stress disorder (PTSD) is a cluster of symptoms that can occur in a person after exposure to a severely stressful event (e.g., rape, combat, natural disaster). There are three categories of symptoms: reexperiencing the event (e.g., nightmares, daydreams, obsessions, flashbacks), withdrawal (e.g., avoiding movies about war and rape and feeling detached from others who have not experienced the event), and hyperarousal (e.g., insomnia, irritability, hypervigilance, severe anxiety). Most patients with PTSD recover, especially those with good premorbid functioning and support. The greatest risk for PTSD among combat veterans is among those who killed noncombatants, participated in atrocities, or were wounded. Another factor associated with increased risk for PTSD is violence or behavioral problems, sociopathy, or psychiatric disorders prior to the trauma. Substance abuse, including alcoholism, is also relevant. It is estimated that as many as 480,000 American veterans of the war in Vietnam have PTSD.

114. The answer is B. *(Kaplan, 7/e, pp 745–746.)* The rigid defensive style characteristic of persons who have obsessive-compulsive neurosis is accomplished by the mechanisms of isolation, undoing, and reaction formation. Isolation is the exclusion of an event from the continuum of meaningful experience; for example, an idea or action may be separated from its original emotional content. Undoing connotes the repetitive patterns of ideation and behavior that are typical of obsessive rituals; an affected patient may feel compelled to undertake an action that counteracts an idea that has recently been expressed or an event that has just occurred. Reaction formation refers to the way in which obsessive-compulsive patients attempt to control an unacceptable wish by undertaking an exaggerated opposing action; kindly actions, for example, may be a reaction against sadistic wishes. In learning theory, obsessions can represent a conditioned stimulus to anxiety so that formerly neutral objects or thoughts become conditioned stimuli that are able to trigger anxiety or discomfort. In compulsion, a certain action is found to reduce anxiety; thus, avoidance strategies (compulsions or rituals) are developed to control the anxieties.

115.   The answer is D. *(Isselbacher, 13/e, pp 2400–2413.)* Anxiety symptoms are very common in both medically ill patients and those otherwise well. In terms of inpatients, 5 to 20 percent have anxiety symptoms and 4 to 14 percent of general medical outpatients suffer from anxiety states. Patients with anxiety disorders are more likely to seek help from general physicians and to use emergency room services than are patients with other types of mental disorders. Furthermore, it has been documented that over the past 15 years, antianxiety medications have been the most frequently prescribed medication in the U.S. Also, primary physicians write over 80 percent of these prescriptions. In terms of other mental disorders, 5.1 percent of the U.S. population suffers from mood disorders—including major depressive, bipolar, and dysthymic—yet they are less apt to seek medical help. Panic disorders occur in 1 to 2 percent of the population and 29 percent of these persons seek help from emergency room services. Obsessive-compulsive disorder usually begins in adolescence or young adulthood, but is not often recognized by general physicians. Help is not often sought because of the private nature of the disorder.

116.   The answer is A. *(Kaplan, 7/e, pp 247–248.)* According to Freud, the superego is the conscience and develops in the ego with the resolution of the Oedipus complex. The conscience refers to the set of internalized moral prohibitions that guides personal behavior. Children build identifications with heroes, teachers, and admired persons in order to form their moral standards, values, aspirations, and ideals. The ego maintains a relationship to the outside world through a sense of reality, reality testing, and adaptation to the reality.

117.   The answer is A. *(Williams, RB, pp 194–197.)* Among the psychosocial variables considered to be risk factors for coronary heart disease, the type A, or coronary-prone, behavior pattern is most prominent. The type A behavior pattern consists of extremes of competitiveness, a chronic sense of time urgency, easily evoked hostility, aggressiveness, explosive speech, and increased rate of activity. More recent studies have shown that aggressiveness and hostility (especially unexpressed hostility) are the most consistent and important factors.

118.   The answer is E. *(Simons, 3/e, pp 48–52.)* Of the psychological defense mechanisms listed, denial is the most common. Most defense mechanisms involve an unconscious mental process and are protective measures for the relief of anxiety or guilt. In denial, the patient attempts to reject the threat of the perception of illness and the developing anxiety. While failure to face one's illness can be harmful, denial can also be a useful defense mechanism, especially during recovery or rehabilitation. In rationalization, a patient attempts to justify an irrational feeling, behavior, or thought. Projection involves attributing one's own problem or conflict to another person or situation. In displacement, a feeling, thought, wish, or fear that is unacceptable is transferred to another person or situation. Sublimation is a defense mechanism whereby wishes that are unacceptable are diverted into acceptable channels; thus partial gratification is achieved. Of the many defense mechanisms, denial is exceeded in frequency only by regression, whereby an illness causes a person to return, in part, to earlier patterns of adapting and behaving.

119. The answer is D. *(Sierles, pp 266–269.)* Between 0.5 and 3 percent of the population experience many vague and fluctuating symptoms in multiple organ systems over time. They are explored with medical tests and treated, but are never "cured." The unexplained symptoms can start in childhood, and the disorder is usually diagnosed by 25 years of age. The *Diagnostic and Statistical Manual of Mental Disorders* (DSM) lists 59 relevant symptoms from multiple organ systems, and a diagnosis of somatization disorder (SD) can be made if a patient experiences at least 13 medically unexplained symptoms from the list. The symptoms have to concern the patient enough to take prescribed medication, to change behavior (e.g., to miss work), or to consult a physician. Episodes of symptoms, sometimes intense, typically last 6 to 9 months, with less intense, but continuing symptoms for 9 to 12 months. Generally, SD is a lifelong condition, and patients with SD consider themselves to be sick. Eighty-six percent report that their symptoms are so disabling that their work is limited. Seventy-five percent are not employed full-time, as compared with 33 percent of patients with other psychiatric diagnoses. When compared with the general population, they are more likely to visit doctors, be hospitalized, and receive unnecessary surgery. Eighty to 90 percent report past depression, 27 percent have hysterectomies for non-cancer-related causes, 17 to 25 percent have irritable bowel syndrome, and 12 percent are chronic pain patients. They are also at increased risk for panic disorder, phobias, general anxiety disorder, obsessive-compulsive disorder, and alcoholism and 47 percent have coexisting personality disorders (avoidant, paranoid, and histrionic). Female-to-male ratios between 2:1 and 20:1 have been reported. There is often an inability to identify and articulate their emotions, they have difficulty habituating to stimuli, and they receive positive reinforcement from medical attention. No treatment cures SD, but patients can be taught about SD and taught a relaxation procedure. Patients should establish regular doctor visits (versus responding to symptoms). Physicians should direct conversation to the patient's personal life and a healthy lifestyle, while deemphasizing symptoms and praising tolerance for symptoms.

120. The answer is C. *(Sierles, pp 125–126.)* The most frequent (about 50 percent) postpartum disorder is a self-limited condition known as postpartum blues, with rapid swings of mood and irritability, decreased concentration, and tearing. Next is postpartum major depression (occasionally mania) in about 10 percent, but most severe is postpartum psychosis (about 1 to 2 per 1000) beginning about 2 to 3 weeks after childbirth. It is still not clear whether postpartum psychosis is a discrete condition or an affective or schizophrenia-like condition precipitated by postpartum stress or endocrine changes. Postpartum psychiatric disorders respond favorably to treatment and have a good prognosis, but in all women who experience a postpartum depression, there is a suicide rate of 5 percent, an infanticide rate of 4 percent, and a recurrence rate of 25 percent for postpartum psychosis and depression after subsequent pregnancies.

121. The answer is D. *(Kaplan, 7/e, pp 229, 258.)* Although Sigmund Freud is best known for the development of the theory of the unconscious, Henry Murray also strongly emphasized the unconscious in the development of his theory of personality. Both Freud and Murray constructed a system of human needs and wishes that existed in the unconscious part of the mind. According to the theory, these unconscious needs and wishes express themselves through the personality and exert considerable influence on individual behavior. Freud arrived at his discovery through the observation of his patients and the analysis of his own dreams, from which he developed his technique of dream analysis. Murray applied the concept of the unconscious in his theory of personality. He is best known for his development of the thematic apperception test, which uses a projective technique to elicit personal and interpersonal conflicts, needs, and attitudes. Carl Jung also placed a strong emphasis on unconscious factors in personality. B. F. Skinner and Kurt Lewin deemphasized the unconscious in the normal personality. Skinner provided experimental analyses of operant behavior to demonstrate that personality is the result of reinforcement and conditioning. Lewin constructed a field theory of action and emotion modeled on physical theory and topology. Margaret Mead had confidence in the psychodynamic unconscious as developed by Freud, but she is best known for her studies demonstrating the importance of cultural mores in molding personality.

122. The answer is B. *(Kaplan, 7/e, p 232.)* The Bender-Gestalt test can be useful in the assessment of maturation and of brain damage. Various atypical responses to the Rorschach cards (e.g., poor form responses) have been found also to be related to brain damage. The Bender-Gestalt test consists of nine test figures that a subject is asked to copy; difficulties in this easy task often are indicative of brain dysfunction. Neither the thematic apperception test nor the California personality inventory has been found to be a sensitive indicator of cerebral damage. The MMPI tests a wide range of personality factors and the MBHI is a psychodiagnostic inventory of personality, coping style, and symptoms for the physically ill. Other than a few cognitive factors, neither is adequate for the detection of brain damage. A frequently used test for brain damage is the Halstead-Reitan battery of neuropsychological tests.

123. The answer is B. *(Gatchel, 2/e, pp 186–187.)* The most usual kinds of compliances are prevention, taking of medication, and alteration in life-style. Medication treatment has an alarmingly low level of compliance and prevention has the lowest. Compliance with chemotherapy for cancer is very high— better than 90 percent. Medication treatment for hypertension, glaucoma, coronary heart disease, and diabetes achieves from 40 to 70 percent compliance from the patient.

124. The answer is C. *(Kaplan, 7/e, pp 249–252.)* Coping mechanisms are actions that resolve conflicts in socially or personally desirable and effective ways. Conflicts are often the results of inconsistencies that exist in our behaviors, our cognitions, or between conflicting cognitions and behaviors. If we are capable of coping, we take action to resolve the problem as well as we can and see that it does not occur again. For example, if there is a conflict between two behaviors, resolution may require considering the behaviors in relationship to our ideals and then changing one or both of them. Or, if the conflict is between two cognitions, we may need to seek information, then pursue changing one or both of the cognitions. If the conflict is between cognition and behavior, then we generally attempt to change either or both to make one conform with the other. Thus coping involves a resolution of the conflict achieved by changing one or both of the conflicting elements. This is not to be confused with the use of defense mechanisms to resolve conflicts. Although defense mechanisms can be appropriate or at least preferable to other available alternatives, they generally "defend" us and do not generally change behavior or resolve the conflict itself. Coping mechanisms confront the problem directly, continue to generate possible solutions, generate more information, get help when needed, and allow us consciously to drop certain habits or form new ones. They allow us to take action to eliminate the undesirable cognition or behavior causing the conflict. Defense mechanisms are most often driven by unconscious forces, such as repression of threatening impulses or ideas, and tend to remove awareness of the conflict. They allow the conflicting elements to continue and provide an illusion of solution, but the problem continues.

125. The answer is B. *(Sierles, pp 103–104.)* Persons with a strong sense of an external locus of health control delegate responsibility for their health to an external force, such as fate, powerful others, chance, or God. They can be relied on to follow treatment orders in the hospital, where they are in an authoritarian system, but as outpatients they cannot be relied on to take responsibility for their own care. They prefer to make as few decisions as possible about their own health and prefer to accept the authority and orders of their own physician, except if the authority is not present to follow up on them. Patients with a strong sense of internal control tend to accept responsibility for and control their own health. This information can be of help to physicians by allowing them to establish follow-up procedures that will insure maximum compliance.

126. The answer is A. *(Sierles, pp 103–104.)* The locus of control regarding health deals with patients' perception of the forces that control their own health. With the perception of an internal locus of control, patients view themselves as being in charge of their own health, take direct responsibility themselves, and consider themselves and their physician to be a team. While physicians often promote this shared responsibility in order to improve compliance, they must recognize and deal with the tendency of those patients to make their own adjustments in the prescribed diet, drug dosage, exercise, or other parts of the regimen. In external locus of control, patients view their health as being controlled by fate, chance, or some other power or authority.

127. The answer is D. *(Simons, 3/e, pp 6–7.)* When people become ill, they become anxious and feel vulnerable to the disease process. They lose a part of their sense of control and autonomy and often become dependent on others, especially if they seek help. The anxiety, dependence, helplessness, and vulnerability will reawaken feelings and recollections of relationships of early childhood and previous life experiences. Their reactions to the illness and to those who are caring for them will be influenced by the way in which they were cared for previously, especially when they were young.

128. The answer is C. *(Hazzard, 3/e, pp 110–111.)* There is much conventional wisdom about how personality changes over the life span, especially during midlife crises and retirement, and how dormant aspects of personality emerge in late life, but the data show otherwise. Studies of adolescents who are followed into adulthood do show somewhat lower levels of stability during adolescence, but there is still considerable continuity in personality from childhood on throughout life. By age 30, both men and women have attained their adult personality, which remains stable with little or no change. While some people experience the legendary midlife crisis, most often this phenomenon takes the form of concern over career choice, physical decline, or discontent with marriage; it is a crisis for only a relatively small portion of middle-aged persons and does not usually result in a personality change. The personality traits of neuroticism, extraversion, openness, agreeableness, and conscientiousness are remarkably stable over time, with the exception that persons with high levels of neuroticism seem to be predisposed to having crises at all ages. Since personality affects health perceptions and health behaviors, it is important that physicians be able to assess and predict the interaction of personality and the patient's reactions to health, illness, and treatment.

129. The answer is A. *(Simons, 3/e, pp 73–78.)* Hypochondriasis is usually characterized as a generalized chronic expression of emotional conflicts through physical symptoms. Such patients are often depressed and may have dependent personalities rather than the histrionic or hysterical personalities seen in patients with conversion disorder. They have a long history of multiple complaints rather than a specific anesthesia or paralysis, and they are usually anxious and worried rather than indifferent. Hypochondriacal patients have a chronic reaction to stress as a "way of life" rather than an acute reaction, and they rarely improve quickly, while a patient with conversion disorder may respond suddenly to treatment.

130. The answer is A. *(Isselbacher, 13/e, p 450.)* Many studies have shown that obese persons respond less well than do normal persons to internal cues, such as gastric contraction. They also overrespond to external cues such as the taste, smell, attractiveness, abundance, and accessibility of food. This is significant because behavior modification can be used to influence eating behaviors by changing the exposure to and pattern and nature of the external cues. Since behavior patterns are learned, they can be changed or unlearned.

131. The answer is E. *(Hazzard, 3/e, pp 109–111.)* Theorists have postulated that the universal processes of aging include the decline of emotionality, the reversal of sex-role-linked characteristics, and the development of wisdom. Longitudinal studies, however, have shown that a person's personality shows little or no change with age. There is little or no change in traits such as emotional stability, sociability, assertiveness, and other characteristics of the individual personality. In other words, a 40 year old who is well adjusted, assertive, and liberal is apt to be a well-adjusted, assertive, liberal 80 year old; likewise, a 40-year-old person who is neurotic and selfish is apt to be a neurotic and selfish 80 year old. Wisdom does appear to increase with age because of experience and education. This is consistent with Erik Erikson's final stage of human development—one attains either integrity or despair.

132. The answer is E. *(Gatchel, 2/e, pp 190–192.)* The health belief model is based on three components of predicting one's compliance behavior: the patient's perceived readiness to act or perception that action is necessary, an estimation of costs and benefits of compliance, and the need for a cue to action, i.e., for an indication that something is wrong. The health belief model takes into account the patient's subjective state or belief regarding his or her health, rather than the objective characteristics of it. The costs and benefits are emphasized, as the patient must believe that the treatment will be effective; i.e., the benefits must outweigh the costs in terms of side effects, disruptiveness, and unpleasantness. The patient's readiness to comply is important, either in terms of internal signals such as pain or discomfort, or external stimuli such as screening programs, costs, and benefits. The health belief model also considers that the patient's perception of the severity of an illness is much more predictive of compliance than is the actual severity of the illness as defined by the doctor or other data.

133. The answer is C. *(Lerner, Psychology, pp 418–419, 514–516.)* Carl Rogers's formulation of client-centered therapy requires that therapists establish an atmosphere of emphatic understanding and of unconditional positive regard for their clients by communicating to them that they are liked and respected whatever they may say or do. Once this atmosphere is established, Rogers's main therapeutic technique is to reflect clients' feelings back to the clients. Rogers feels that this helps them to clarify feelings and attitudes that are conflictive or otherwise difficult. He further argues that a client-centered therapist should not offer interpretations of behavior, attitudes, or unconscious wishes and feelings.

134. The answer is E. *(Kaplan, 7/e, pp 223–227.)* Projective methods of personality assessment comprise those measures that are relatively unstructured and have no correct answers. Subjects' responses to such measures are presumed to be more indicative of individual characteristics than is the case with more structured tests, responses to which are inclined to be determined more by the nature of the test than of the subject taking it. The thematic apperception test, draw-a-person test, sentence completion test, and Rorschach test are all considered to be projective methods of measurement. The Minnesota multiphasic personality inventory (MMPI) is a structured personality inventory of 550 items that must be answered "True, " "False," or "Cannot Say."

135. The answer is B. *(Sierles, pp 142–143.)* There are over 250,000 reported cases of sexual abuse each year, yet except for physical signs of genital or anal trauma, STD, or recurrent urinary tract or vaginal infections, the physician (or family) has very few methods of securing supporting evidence, especially in the younger child. Frequently, certain behavioral manifestations can be of assistance. These may include a child's simulation of sex acts with dolls, the inclusion of genitalia in drawings, veiled verbal references to molestation, occasional sleep or appetite disorders, or even phobias relating to being touched (e.g., during bathing) or reacting against a certain person or room. Depression and suicidal behavior can also develop in an older child. Hugging and body touching of others is more often decreased rather than increased. The most frequent intrafamilial abusers of girls are uncles, stepfathers, fathers, first cousins, and brothers.

136. The answer is B. *(Isselbacher, 13/e, pp 2414–2417.)* Schizophrenia is a serious mental disorder with about 1 percent prevalence across all cultures. It has a 6-month or longer duration and causes significant social, occupational, and personal disability and suffering. Diagnosis includes at least 6 months of bizarre delusions often with persecutory or jealous content, auditory hallucinations, and grossly disorganized behavior. The most significant etiologic factor is genetic as confirmed by twin, family, and adoption studies. There is a higher incidence in persons of lower socioeconomic status, but it is difficult to determine whether this is because of a "social drift" of more vulnerable persons or the stresses of lower socioeconomic status, especially in genetically vulnerable persons. A major psychosocial factor is a frequent pattern of communication conflicts between parents and between parents and the child or developing adult. There is also a stress-diathesis model whereby predisposed persons are vulnerable to certain stressful circumstances. The phenothiazines are the most effective form of chemical treatment.

137. The answer is C. *(Kaplan, 7/e, pp 824–828.)* Before the development of psychoanalytic theory, psychopathologic manifestations were considered to be evidence of mental disorders having nothing in common with normal mental functioning. One of Freud's greatest contributions lay in his recognition that the same psychological processes operate in both normal and abnormal mental functioning, i.e., that any differences between normality and abnormality are quantitative, not qualitative. The necessary implication of Freud's perception is that any judgments as to a person's "normality" are relative and that there are no absolute criteria by which a person can be classified as psychologically ill.

138. The answer is D. *(Kaplan, 7/e, pp 573–578.)* There is no simple linear relationship between task performance and level of arousal or anxiety. The Yerkes-Dodson theory posits a curvilinear relationship between these variables in which performance is enhanced at a certain optimal level of arousal; anxiety levels lower or higher than this optimum have a detrimental effect on performance. There is evidence in support of the Yerkes-Dodson formulation. It also has been demonstrated that such factors as task complexity, instructional set, and intelligence alter the quantitative features of the curvilinear relationship between performance and anxiety.

139–142. The answers are 139-E, 140-C, 141-A, 142-B. *(Kaplan, 7/e, pp 221–236.)* The Bender-Gestalt test is a test of visual motor coordination and is useful in both children and adults. Initially it was used as a measure of a child's maturational level, according to how many of the nine designs a child could reproduce at various levels of accuracy. It is now used most frequently with adults as a screening device for signs of organic brain dysfunction. It can also be used in assessing mental retardation, aphasias, psychoses, neuroses, and malingering.

The Minnesota multiphasic personality inventory, an objective self-report test to assess personality, is one of the most widely used tests for clinical and research purposes. It provides scores on ten clinical scales: hypochondriasis (Hs), depression (D), hysteria (Hy), psychopathic deviation (Pd), masculinity-femininity (Mf), paranoia (Pa), psychasthenia (Pt), schizophrenia (Sc), hypomania (Ma), and social distance (Si); plus three additional scales: a lie scale (L) to detect attempts to present oneself in a good light, a frequency scale (F) of unconventional beliefs and attitudes, and a correction scale (K) for guardedness or defensiveness in test-taking. The MMPI, like all tests, is most effectively used in conjunction with other information about the patient. It is currently being restandardized based on a contemporary sample of normal people.

The Halstead-Reitan battery of neurologic tests was developed in the early 1940s to determine the location and effects of specific brain lesions. It is composed of ten tests: category test (to identify common elements in a set of pictures for concept function, abstraction, and visual acuity), tactual performance test, rhythm test, finger-oscillation test, speech-sounds perception test, trial-making test, critical flicker frequency, time sense test, aphasia screening test, and sensory-perception test. The usefulness of the Halstead-Reitan battery can be enhanced by using it in conjunction with the MMPI and the Wechsler adult intelligence scale.

The Wechsler adult intelligence scale (WAIS) is the best standardized test of intelligence in use today. There are six verbal subtests and five performance subtests and it yields a verbal IQ, a performance IQ, and a combined IQ. The eleven subtests are general information, comprehension (proverbs), arithmetic, similarities (between two things), digit-span (recall of two to nine digits), vocabulary (definitions), picture completion (with a missing part), block design (matched color and designs), picture arrangements (arrange series to tell a story), object assembly (organize objects in order), and digit symbol (pair symbols with digits). There is also a scale for children ages 5 through 15, and a preschool version for ages 4 to $6\frac{1}{2}$ years.

The thematic apperception test (TAT), designed by Henry Murray and Christiana Morgan in 1943, has 30 pictures with ambiguity in each picture. The subject creates a story about each picture that reveals approach to organization, sequence, vocabulary, style, preconceptions, assumptions, and outcome. It is especially useful for inferring motivational aspects of behavior rather than as a diagnostic test.

143–145. The answers are 143-A, 144-D, 145-C. *(Kaplan, 7/e, pp 249–252.)* Reaction formation is the defensive process whereby an unacceptable feeling or impulse is converted into, and consciously experienced as, its opposite. Thus, in reaction formation, "I hate him" becomes "I love him."

Projection is the process through which unacceptable impulses are at once denied and attributed to someone else or to something in the environment. Thus, in projection, "I hate him" is converted into "he hates me."

Denial is the defense mechanism by means of which any aspect of reality, e.g., forbidden thoughts, is actively denied. With this defense mechanism, "I hate him" becomes "I don't hate him."

The defense mechanism of undoing refers to an action that is meant somehow to reverse or "undo" the damage that is felt to have been caused by an unacceptable wish.

Isolation is the conscious experience of an unacceptable wish or thought without the painful effect associated with it. Isolation and undoing both are defenses characteristic of people who have obsessive-compulsive personality styles.

146–149. The answers are 146-C, 147-A, 148-B, 149-D. *(Plomin, 2/e, pp 349–354.)* Dizygotic (fraternal) twins have similar but not identical genes. The similarity of their genes, however, is not significantly greater than that of other siblings. The fact that the IQs of fraternal twins reared in the same environment are more alike (correlation coefficient: 0.60) than those of other siblings reared in similar circumstances (0.47) must reflect experiential influences on IQ.

The highest correlation between IQ scores is obtained from monozygotic (identical) twins. Identical twins reared together have a correlation coefficient of 0.86; those reared apart, 0.72. This high correlation may be assumed to be a result of both hereditary and environmental factors. In fact, since monozygotic twins have identical genomes, it may be argued that an even higher correlation would exist were it not for the unavoidable factor of slight differences in experience.

The correlation between IQs of siblings reared together (0.47) is higher than that for siblings reared apart (0.24). This observation seems to suggest that environmental factors affect IQ scores considerably. The fact that there is a significant correlation between IQs of siblings reared apart demonstrates the contribution of hereditary factors to intelligence.

A relatively high correlation appears between the IQ scores of siblings reared together. It is much lower, however, than the correlation between dizygotic twins, although their genomes are about equally heterogeneous. This difference is probably attributable to the fact that both society and families tend to treat twins more alike than they do other siblings.

The lowest observed correlation between IQs of offspring occurs for siblings reared apart. However, the correlation is significantly higher than that for unrelated persons who are reared together. Thus it seems that hereditary factors are somewhat more potent determinants of IQ than either environmental or experiential factors.

150–152. The answers are 150-B, 151-A, 152-E. *(Gatchel, 2/e, pp 39–49.)* The medical profession has been concerned with stress for centuries. Hippocrates spoke of suffering caused by disease (*pathos*), but separated it from the toil involved in resisting and fighting disease (*ponos*). He thus suggested a stresslike aspect of illness.

Walter Cannon suggested that stress had both physiologic and psychological components in response to danger. He is most famous for his description of the sympathetic nervous system acting to ready a threatened organism for "fight or flight" by producing a heightened state of arousal. Stress can aid in survival, but it can also disrupt emotional and physiologic stability (homeostasis). Thus, emotional stress could cause physiologic disturbances that lead to medical problems.

Hans Selye developed the general adaptation syndrome (GAS), which consisted of three stages: the alarm reaction, the stage of resistance, and the stage of exhaustion. The presence of a noxious stimulus or stressor causes an alarm reaction in preparation for resisting the stressor. When the body reserves are mobilized, the stage of resistance applies various physiologic and psychological coping mechanisms to adapt or fend off the stressor, but usually with a decrease in resistance to other stimuli or threats. When these reactions are repeated many times or over a prolonged time, the stage of exhaustion is reached and the organism is at risk for irreversible physiologic damage. With reserves depleted and resistance no longer possible, the wear and tear and exhaustion then lead to the onset of diseases of adaptation, such as kidney disease, arthritis, and cardiovascular disease.

John Mason and Marianne Frankenhauser extended Selye's GAS into the psychosocial realm. They postulated that stress is more than a reaction to nonspecific stimuli and that some kind of psychological awareness of noxious or stressful events may be necessary for stress to occur. More importantly, they demonstrated that psychological factors can actually alter bodily functioning and lead to illness. These and other findings have established an important link between psychosocial factors and health.

Richard Lazarus recognized the significance of psychological stress. In order for an event to evoke a stressful reaction, it must be appraised by the individual as threatening. This allows one to evaluate the dangers and benefits of the stressful event, select a coping option, and even reappraise the event as it evolves. Personality, experience, and goals can also affect the interpretation. Thus, the same event can be interpreted by one person as a threat and by another as a challenge. Lazarus also postulated that daily problems can be just as important in causing stress as less frequent but more severe threats.

153–155. The answers are 153-E, 154-D, 155-A. *(Gatchel, 2/e, pp 105–112. Ragland, N Engl J Med 318: 65–69, 1988.)* Sir William Osler (1892) observed that the typical coronary patient was robust, keen and ambitious, vigorous in mind and body, and one "whose engine is always at full speed ahead." In the late 1950s Richard Rosenman and Milton Friedman described the type A behavior pattern and developed a reliable technique for its assessment. They characterized the type A behaviors as excessive competitive drive, impatience, hostility, and vigorous speech. The type B person was considered to possess a relative lack of these characteristics and have a more easygoing style of coping. Rosenman and Friedman developed a structured interview focused on observable behavior based on speech characteristics and how persons responded to questions rather than how they described themselves.

David Jenkins in the early 1970s developed the Jenkins Activity Survey (JAS). The JAS is a questionnaire relying on a person's report of his or her own behavior. It is still frequently used as a clinical screening measure as well as a research tool.

David Glass emphasized that the type A pattern should be considered more as a coping style used to establish and maintain control over stressful situations. Type A persons respond to stress or to a challenge by accelerating the pace of their work and by becoming more competitive, aggressive, or hostile. He found that type A persons respond to uncontrollable stress or situations by working harder or faster than do type B persons. Also, they perceive challenges as more threatening, which arouses a sense of urgency, competitiveness, hostility, and a greater physiologic response with increased sympathetic arousal and secretion of epinephrine and norepinephrine.

Karen Mathews explored the genesis of type A behavior in one's early years, as early as age 5. She developed the Mathews Youth Test for Health, which is completed by an observer of a child's behavior. Mathews has demonstrated type A and type B patterns of behavior in children as young as age 9 and has recently developed a scale for adolescents. She has found that the behaviors of achievement, anger-arousal, and impulsiveness are stable from about 6 to 10 years of age to adulthood and that these type A children experience the same elevations in heart rate and blood pressure in response to psychological challenges as do their adult counterparts.

D. R. Ragland and R. J. Brand in a recent study (1988) found that if one studies persons who have already survived a coronary event, the type B patients are more apt to suffer a subsequent coronary event than are their type A counterparts. While this does not negate the increased risk of type A persons for the initial coronary event, it does raise the question of other interactive factors; for example, type A patients may respond differently than type B patients to a coronary event. Type A patients may be better able to cope, comply with treatment, change life-style, and so on, and thus improve their prognosis.

156–159. The answers are 156-C, 157-E, 158-I, 159-H. *(Sierles, pp 272–274.)* Persons with a paranoid personality disorder are suspicious, hypervigilant, and preoccupied with others' fidelity and often perceive themselves as righteous and others as corrupt. The warehouse clerk could be expressing hostility by projecting or rationalizing his own behavior as a kind of righteous defense against a boss whom he chooses to label a robber. The prevalence of paranoid personality disorder is not known, but there is some evidence that there is a heritable link with delusional disorder and schizophrenia. Psychotherapy and perhaps a low dose of antipsychotic medication to relieve anxiety will help, although many patients will not take any medication.

A person with an antisocial personality is considered a sociopath who is callous, lacks remorse or guilt, is often cruel to animals, and is selfish. These persons can be very sociable with a superficial charm (which can make them excellent "con artists"), but they become irritable and resentful if their needs are not met or if they do not get their way. Antisocial personality disorder begins in childhood and continues throughout life. The life expectancy of those with this disorder is shortened by accidents, homicide, and the consequences of substance abuse. In childhood they are often truant, run away from home, fight, vandalize, lie, and rob with confrontation of the victim. As adults, they avoid working, abandon jobs, fight, abuse or neglect family, malinger, and engage in reckless behavior. Three-fourths of convicted felons have antisocial personalities. They often feel that their behavior is justified because of the alleged mistreatment to which they have been subjected. These patients are difficult to treat with psychotherapy because of their self-destructive behavior.

Persons with borderline personality disorder have an intense intolerance for feeling alone. They act dramatically and can be self-destructive. The student on the balcony took dramatic action, which provoked a rescue that could be taken as the rescuer's love. Persons with borderline personality disorder are unstable, idealize love, erupt violently at times, and have moods that range widely from boredom or emptiness to rage. Mood disorders are common in their families. Psychotherapy or a combination of psychotherapy and pharmacotherapy is standard treatment.

A person with a passive-aggressive personality disorder demonstrates covert noncompliance, especially with authority. The bookkeeper's forgetting, procrastinating, and arriving late can be a passive way to express aggression in response to anger and frustration. Psychotherapy is the treatment of choice.

Learning and Behavioral Change

DIRECTIONS: Each question below contains five suggested responses. Select the **one best** response to each question.

160. A behavior pattern that increases in frequency when followed by a reward is an example of

(A) classical conditioning
(B) shaping
(C) respondent conditioning
(D) operant conditioning
(E) generalization

161. In operant conditioning, the rate of extinction is most effectively slowed when the response or learning has been maintained on a reinforcement schedule of

(A) fixed ratio
(B) variable ratio
(C) fixed interval reinforcement
(D) continuous reinforcement
(E) piecework reinforcement

162. The idea that experimental extinction, which is produced by nonreinforcement after classical conditioning, is an active inhibitory process finds support in the phenomenon of

(A) generalization
(B) spontaneous recovery
(C) experimental neurosis
(D) passive avoidance
(E) active avoidance

163. Which of the following behavioral methods of treating asthma has proved to be most effective when combined with medical treatment?

(A) Psychotherapy
(B) Behavioral self-management
(C) Psychoanalysis
(D) Employment of suggestion strategies
(E) Diminishment of emotional reactions

164. In classical conditioning, the "partial reinforcement effect" is the

(A) inability to learn with fractional reward
(B) increased response retention following partial reinforcement
(C) increased conditional response amplitudes after nonreinforced trials
(D) reduced response latencies on nonreinforced trials
(E) contrast effects for partial reinforcement schedules

165. A major distinction between the methods for producing classical and instrumental conditioning is that in instrumental conditioning the reinforcing stimulus is

(A) always appetitive in nature
(B) contingent on the behavior to be learned
(C) invariant
(D) solely under the control of the experimenter
(E) unnecessary to produce learning

166. The term *learning disabilities* most often refers to problems in learning

(A) to do arithmetic
(B) to read
(C) to write compositions
(D) eye-hand coordination
(E) achievement orientation

167. The most important component of biofeedback is

(A) feelings
(B) information
(C) motivation
(D) attitude
(E) interpersonal relations

168. In educational programs designed to limit the spread of HIV infection, which of the following intervention strategies has been most effective in producing behavioral change?

(A) Provision of health education
(B) Random testing of a person's knowledge of AIDS
(C) Recruitment to an STD clinic program
(D) Use of peers as endorsers of behavioral change
(E) Appeal to sexual partners to change behavior

169. In patients with cancer who are to receive chemotherapy, behavioral conditioning results in anticipatory nausea in

(A) two-thirds of these patients
(B) the more hopeful and optimistic patients
(C) patients high in chronic anxiety
(D) the more gregarious patients
(E) the less inhibited patients

170. In applying behavioral modification to weight reduction, the most important initial step is to

(A) work with the patient to establish a baseline diet
(B) do a daily caloric intake analysis
(C) begin a mild but systematic exercise program
(D) identify all medications being taken
(E) compile a detailed history of the patient's eating patterns

171. In treatment programs for alcohol dependence, the risk of relapse is increased if the patient is

(A) maintained in an environment free of alcohol-associated stimuli
(B) provided therapeutic strategies to extinguish alcohol-compensatory conditioned responses
(C) returned to an environment different from the one in which the dependence was acquired
(D) provided procedures to extinguish conditioned associations between aversive affective states and alcohol
(E) allowed to substitute the use of other non-alcoholic drugs when negative affective states occur

172. You have just told a patient with a family history of cardiovascular disease to quit smoking. What percentage of the patients given such advice will quit smoking?

(A) 5
(B) 10
(C) 15
(D) 20
(E) 25

173. In B. F. Skinner's view, the study of behavior

(A) should be concerned with the fundamental motives that are found in all organisms
(B) should employ factor-analytic procedures to identify the basic dimensions of personality
(C) must be based entirely on an understanding of classical conditioning
(D) cannot make extrapolations about principles of learning from subhuman species to humans
(E) need not make inferences about unobservable organismic states and inner motives

DIRECTIONS: Each numbered question or incomplete statement below is NEGATIVELY phrased. Select the **one best** lettered response.

174. All the following are basic principles of the neural basis of learning and memory EXCEPT

(A) memory has stages and is continually changing
(B) long-term memory results in physical changes in the brain
(C) memory traces are widely distributed throughout the nervous system
(D) the hippocampus and temporal lobes are most actively involved in the human memory process
(E) localized trauma can completely destroy stored memory

175. In order for operant conditioning to be effectively applied to a psychiatric disorder (e.g., shouting obscenities), one can increase positive, constructive behavior by all the following EXCEPT

(A) precisely defining desired behavior
(B) identifying an effective reinforcer
(C) providing reinforcement when desired behavior is emitted
(D) punishing undesired behavior
(E) exchanging a preferred food for desired behavior

176. Learned helplessness is associated with depression in that both are characterized by each of the following EXCEPT

(A) continued failure from lack of ability
(B) passive behavior
(C) negative expectations
(D) hopelessness
(E) feelings of no control over events

177. Of the following methods of behavioral treatment to reduce blood pressure, which has NOT been found effective?

(A) Biofeedback
(B) Meditation
(C) Contingency conditioning
(D) Relaxation
(E) Weight loss

178. All the following factors are critical in both classical and operant conditioning EXCEPT

(A) timing
(B) stimulus discrimination
(C) specific reflex responses
(D) extinction
(E) learning of predictive relationships

179. A social learning approach to attitude change includes all the following methods EXCEPT

(A) modeling
(B) desensitization
(C) extinction
(D) direct reinforcement
(E) integration of nature (vs. nurture)

180. Correct statements regarding systematic desensitization include all the following EXCEPT

(A) it was developed by Joseph Wolpe
(B) it is used to decrease neurotic anxiety or phobia
(C) anxiety-provoking situations are brought to mind to be resolved through reality therapy
(D) anxiety-provoking situations are paired with anxiety-reducing relaxation
(E) the patient is taught a technique of muscular relaxation

181. All the following strategies for preventing HIV in high-risk persons have proved effective EXCEPT

(A) training of peers as endorsers of behavioral change
(B) making persons aware of their susceptibility and vulnerability
(C) promoting fear and disapproval
(D) promoting information and needle-exchange programs among IV drug users
(E) making persons aware that the benefits of behavior change outweigh the costs

182. Of the following behavioral techniques, the LEAST effective in relieving migraine headaches is

(A) psychotherapy
(B) relaxation training
(C) biofeedback of finger temperature
(D) systematic desensitization
(E) constriction of extracranial arteries

183. In attempting to understand how adolescents develop the habit of smoking, social learning theory cites all the following reasons EXCEPT

(A) lack of learned negative expectations
(B) acquired positive expectations
(C) inhibition
(D) learned behaviors
(E) powers of observation

184. Accurate statements regarding our knowledge of intervention and skills in changing health behavior include all the following EXCEPT

(A) we know a lot about how to help people change initially, but are not as successful at helping them sustain the new behavior
(B) we are not well informed about preparing and motivating people to undertake change
(C) we know more about health promotion than about risk reduction
(D) we know very little about how people successfully change their own behavior without assistance
(E) we know very little about how to assure patient compliance

185. Which of the following strategies of intervention would be LEAST effective in changing a person's type A pattern of behavior?

(A) Changing environmental demands

(B) Changing the patient's response to the environment

(C) Changing physiologic concomitants of type A behavior

(D) Changing the expectations of the social group or society

(E) Progressive relaxation training

186. Social factors that play a major role in influencing junior and senior high school students to smoke include all the following EXCEPT

(A) peer pressure

(B) cigarette advertising

(C) modeling

(D) social inoculation

(E) experimentation

187. Nutritional experts have recommended all the following behavioral tips for weight control EXCEPT

(A) eating slowly

(B) taking small portions of food

(C) waiting 20 minutes before taking a second helping

(D) watching television or reading while you are eating

(E) recording all food intake in a "dietary diary"

188. Physicians can help patients change their health-related behavior patterns by all the following EXCEPT

(A) discovering and responding to the patient's expectations

(B) simplifying the health treatment plan as much as possible

(C) providing the knowledge to support the recommended behavior

(D) instilling a sense of personal responsibility in the patient for his or her own health maintenance

(E) assuring patients that their health maintenance is solely the responsibility of their physicians

189. Fordyce's classic behavioral approach to pain is based on all the following EXCEPT

(A) behavior in response to pain is significant in its own right

(B) environmental consequences have a strong effect on pain-related behavior

(C) pain behavior is observable and measurable

(D) understanding internal causative factors of conflict or anxiety is crucial

(E) operant conditioning mechanisms are involved

190. Environmental influences on pain and pain-related behavior involve all the following learning mechanisms EXCEPT

(A) operant conditioning
(B) classical conditioning
(C) respondent conditioning
(D) observational learning
(E) latent learning

191. Behaviorally conditioned alterations of immune response are demonstrated by all the following EXCEPT

(A) conditioned compensatory responses
(B) conditioned suppression of cell-mediated immune responses
(C) extinction of conditioned suppression of antibody-mediated immune responses
(D) development of tolerance to an immunomodulating agent
(E) conditioning of the immunologic effects of stress

DIRECTIONS: Each group of questions below consists of lettered headings followed by a set of numbered items. For each numbered item select the **one** lettered heading with which it is **most** closely associated. Each lettered heading may be used **once, more than once, or not at all.**

Questions 192–195

Match each description below with the appropriate learning mechanism.

(A) Contact desensitization
(B) Shaping
(C) Systematic desensitization
(D) Operant conditioning
(E) Classical conditioning

192. Pairs a neutral stimulus with a stimulus that produces a known response until the neutral stimulus alone produces the known response

193. Develops new behaviors and increases the probability of a response by introducing reward or reinforcement

194. Typically pairs muscle relaxation with a hierarchy of imagined scenes associated with anxiety

195. Reinforces successive approximations until the desired response is obtained

Questions 196–197

For each description, select the most appropriate learning mechanism.

(A) Negative reinforcement
(B) Modeling
(C) Habituation
(D) Operant conditioning
(E) Classical conditioning

196. A 45-year-old female patient is undergoing regular chemotherapy for her breast cancer; her last visit she became nauseated and vomited as she entered the clinic room

197. A medical student becomes more comfortable in the anatomy laboratory after several weeks of exposure to it

Questions 198–199

For each case, select the most appropriate learning mechanism involved.

(A) Stimulus control
(B) Desensitization
(C) Fixed-interval reinforcement
(D) Variable-ratio reinforcement
(E) Variable-interval reinforcement

198. An obese woman is not losing weight on a weight-loss program and is returning to your office for the monthly checkup; she confesses to not adhering to the program during the first few weeks and then going on a "crash" diet during the week preceding the planned checkup

199. An obese man who is trying to lose weight observes that he enjoys nibbling on certain foods while watching television; you advise him to limit his eating to the kitchen and to refrain from nibbling on anything while watching television

Questions 200–201

For each case, select the most appropriate learning mechanism involved.

(A) Habituation
(B) Aversive conditioning
(C) Stimulus control
(D) Variable-ratio reinforcement
(E) Systematic desensitization

200. In a program aimed at cessation of smoking, a patient is required to smoke many cigarettes in a small booth and over a short period of time

201. A 40-year-old man who works for the state as a highway and bridge designer becomes extremely anxious when he has to drive across any bridge—Which technique can best help him?

Questions 202–205

For each description below, match the appropriate mechanism of behavior change.

(A) Contingency management stimulus control
(B) Cognitive restructuring
(C) Thought-stopping procedures
(D) Self-control techniques
(E) Biofeedback

202. Effective in controlling one's autonomic bodily functions by using visual and auditory cues

203. Effective in changing the frequency of behavior by systematically using reinforcement or the consequences of behavior.

204. Effective in reducing anxiety

205. Effective in reducing obsessions

Learning and Behavioral Change

Answers

160. The answer is D. *(Schneiderman, pp 162–163.)* The influence of behavior by rewards and punishments has its roots in classical studies of learning. In the earlier classical conditioning experiments, Pavlov investigated the acquired associations between environmental stimuli (food, bell) and smooth muscle responses (salivation). By pairing the food and bell, he elicited salivation using only the bell. This is known as generalization of a response to two or more stimuli. In operant conditioning, the desired behavior is rewarded or reinforced with an object, food, praise, or other reward of pleasing consequence to the learner. Shaping involves rewarding the person's behavior as it begins to approach or approximate the desired or ideal behavior until the desired behavior is reached or mastered. The therapeutic use of this ability to increase or control certain behaviors by reinforcing the desired behavior is the essence of behavioral modification. Behavioral modification has repeatedly demonstrated its efficacy in changing behavior and establishing "good" behaviors in such areas as self-care, social behavior, psychiatric pathology, eating behaviors, smoking, and pain.

161. The answer is B. *(Kaplan, 7/e p 166.)* Extinction is the gradual reduction of a conditioned response, usually the result of withholding or altering the reinforcement or reward. Extinction is slowed when reinforcement occurs on a variable schedule (i.e., not every response being rewarded) rather than a continuous reinforcement schedule (every response rewarded). Gambling behavior, for example, is maintained powerfully through variable ratio reinforcement, even when there are long periods of nonreinforced responses. A fixed ratio schedule would provide a reinforcement after a specific number of responses or objects were produced (e.g., in a factory worker's schedule). In a fixed interval schedule, a person is reinforced only after a certain time has elapsed, such as with a monthly salary check. Piecework reinforcement is similar to a fixed ratio schedule with a reward being provided after each piece of work is produced.

162. The answer is B. *(Gatchel, 2/e, pp 217–220.)* Spontaneous recovery, first described by Pavlov, is the return of response strength in due course after extinction. If extinction produced forgetting, then presumably the loss of responsiveness would be permanent. Return of the previously learned material suggests that it is not lost but rather suppressed by some active process resulting from nonreinforcement. Additional support for this concept comes from the finding that responses may return at full strength following a single reinforcement at the end of extinction.

163. The answer is B. *(Linden, pp 221–242.)* Asthma is a very complex respiratory condition. An attack can be triggered or precipitated by a multitude of stimuli and events. The old psychoanalytic explanations and models of several decades ago have been almost completely discredited and even the remaining hope for the efficacy of individual psychotherapeutic treatment lacks sufficient evidence. There is no cure for asthma, but there is considerable evidence that some degree of control can be attained. It is in this context that both sound medical treatment and behavioral self-management can be combined to greatly enhance the control of the disorder. The behavioral self-management program includes education (e.g., mechanics of breathing, use of medications) and self-management training (e.g., self-monitoring and observation of reactions, use of diaries, information processing of own data, decision making with most appropriate options, and self-instruction at all phases of the program). Suggestion can sometimes alter pulmonary function in asthmatic patients, but it has not had adequate success. Even though emotional reactions can act to trigger an asthmatic attack, attempts to eliminate or reduce emotional reactions have proved less effective than self-management in controlling asthma.

164. The answer is B. *(Simons, 3/e, pp 608–610.)* The retarded rate of extinction following partial reinforcement in acquisition was labeled the "partial reinforcement effect" by Lloyd Humphreys (1939). This consistent effect was regarded as something of a paradox since resistance to extinction was thought to be a function of response strength built up by reinforcement during training. According to this reasoning, partial reinforcement should produce faster, not slower, extinction.

165. The answer is B. *(Simons, 3/e, pp 609–610.)* A contingency relationship between response and reinforcement is characteristic of instrumental conditioning. For this form of learning, reinforcement occurs only if the desired response is emitted. Therefore, the occurrence of reinforcement is at least partly under the control of the learner.

166. The answer is B. *(Simons, 3/e, pp 638–646.)* *Learning disability* is the label given to children who show a discrepancy between their estimated academic potential and their actual level of academic performance. Failure to learn academically does not necessarily imply general impairment in intellectual capacity, but it can seriously affect broad adaptive functioning. Most persons with learning disabilities show a largely selective deficit, despite apparently normal schooling exposure, seemingly normative family settings, appropriate motivational predispositions, intact sense organs, adequate physical status, and normal intelligence, yet they fail to learn with normal proficiency. Research studies show that the criterion of failure to learn to read is the most frequent manifestation of a learning disability. This form of learning disability is generally known as dyslexia and is a problem of major proportions, especially during adolescence.

167. The answer is B. *(Gatchel, 2/e, pp 231–234.)* Biofeedback is a process of learning to control various components of one's autonomic responses by using visual or auditory feedback of information from one's physiologic functions. The feedback of information about one's physiologic responses and one's ability to learn and practice control can be influenced by such factors as motivation, feelings, attitude, and interpersonal relations, but information feedback is the primary component in the learning process. Just as one learns to improve one's motor skills by feedback of information and observations of distance, time, space, improvement, and so on, one can learn to exert influence on physiologic responses. Formerly these physiologic responses had been regarded as autonomic because we had no visual electronic or mechanical mechanism for feeding back such information.

168. The answer is D. *(Sierles, p 10.)* One of the most effective methods of changing behavior is through the participation and appeal of popular and influencial leaders. This has been demonstrated in educational programs to prevent sexual transmission of HIV with the use of popular leaders in the male homosexual community who had been trained to serve as endorsers of behavioral change. Anal intercourse was reduced after 2 months from 37 to 28 percent and the proportion of men who had multiple partners was decreased by 18 percent. Intravenous drug users also increased the use of bleach to clean their needles and syringes if they believed their friends and peers did likewise. Such peer leaders have also proved effective in reducing smoking among adolescents.

169. The answer is C. *(Gatchel, 2/e, pp 177–178.)* The behavioral conditioning process is very active in cancer patients who are receiving chemotherapy. The conditioned response of anticipatory nausea occurs because certain personal, environmental, or situational stimuli may elicit nausea before the administration of the chemotherapy that can cause nausea in its own right. About one-third of cancer patients on chemotherapy develop anticipatory nausea. It also occurs more frequently in patients who are less hopeful and more pessimistic, isolated, and inhibited, and those who have more chronic anxiety. The anticipatory nausea also appears to be related to the severity of the dose of chemotherapy. The major stimuli involved can be the hospital, the clinic, the nurse, or the smells encountered before administration of the chemotherapy.

170. The answer is E. *(Isselbacher, 13/e, p 450.)* The most important initial component is to explore and compile a detailed history of the individual patient's eating patterns. It may also be important to analyze the daily caloric intake, establish a diet, begin an exercise program, and identify current medications, but these are not initial concerns. The history should identify (and document when possible) such eating patterns as time of day, length of eating period, place of eating (kitchen, television room, dining room, in front of stove or refrigerator), whether the patient stands or sits while eating, simultaneous activities (watching television, reading, dressing), emotional state, companions (relatives, friends, alone), the kinds and quantities of foods eaten, and dieting practices in the past (successful and unsuccessful). Once the eating practices are known, an individualized strategy for behavioral change can be developed (with the patient) designed to disrupt or abolish certain patterns that initiate or prolong "unhealthy" practices and substitute behavioral changes that will promote weight loss. Emotional states frequently affect eating, especially if food is used as a pacifier. For example, in behavioral modification, one practices the substitution of other activities when the patient recognizes the occurrence of a vulnerable emotional state. The success of this strategy is gauged by its identification and modification of patterns of eating and the long-term maintenance of improved patterns of eating and physical activity.

171. The answer is E. *(Linden, pp 27–29.)* Evaluations of treatment methods using the classical conditioning model have demonstrated that relapse is more likely to occur in the presence of alcohol-associated stimuli. Thus, the most effective treatment conditions should maintain an environment that is as free as possible of alcohol-associated stimuli, and the patient should be returned to an environment that is different from the one in which dependence was acquired. Since dependence is acquired by the patient's developing alcohol-compensatory conditioned responses, specific, therapeutic strategies should be implemented and practiced over time prior to discharge in order to extinguish these alcohol-compensatory conditioned responses. Aversive affective states, such as depression or anxiety, can also act to increase the likelihood of relapse, so all treatment procedures should attempt to extinguish conditioned associations between aversive affective states and alcohol. The patient will probably experience relief from withdrawal symptoms if allowed to substitute other drugs; thus the very conditioned responses targeted for extinction will be maintained.

172. The answer is B. *(Sierles, pp 79–81.)* Even though most smokers say that they would try to quit smoking if their physician told them to quit, only a third even try and only 10 percent actually do quit. Studies show that two-thirds of smokers have not been told by their physicians to quit or even to smoke less, although the number of physicians giving such advice is increasing. However, it is still considered good advice, even with a 10 percent success rate, since this still adds up to a significant number of people who actually quit. There are now several excellent behaviorally based programs for cessation of smoking that the physician can recommend and monitor.

173. The answer is E. *(Kaplan, 7/e, p 259.)* B. F. Skinner's radical behaviorist approach to psychology is based on the idea that the behavioral sciences should be restricted to the recording and analysis of *observable* behavioral responses. Skinner argued that it is unnecessary to make inferences about such inner states as arousal, need levels, motives, and cognitions. Skinner analyzed behavior in terms of the principles of classic Pavlovian conditioning and, more importantly, operant learning. Operant learning (instrumental conditioning) involves changing the relationship between reinforcement schedules and response outcomes.

174. The answer is E. *(Kandel, 3/e, pp 997–1007).* Memory can be divided into short-term and long-term stages. Recently acquired memories are more easily disrupted by such factors as trauma, whereas long-term memories, or older memories, are fairly resistant to disturbance. Short-term memory is transformed into a more permanent long-term store. Thus, the memory process is always undergoing continual change with time. Both short-term and long-term memories are encoded in neural activity that involves a physical change in the brain with apparent alterations of the connections between neurons. It is also clear that the memory traces are not localized to any one brain structure, and that all parts of the nervous system have the plastic properties needed for memory storage. The recall involves an active reconstruction rather than a faithful reproduction of the internal store, and the complex nature of learning itself ensures that the involved neurons are widely distributed in the nervous system. Fortunately, the brain has the capacity to take limited remaining information (memory) and reconstruct a relatively good reproduction of the original memory. The temporal lobes and associated areas and the hippocampus are not registers or banks for memory storage but are actively involved in the storage and retrieval process. Since memory traces are not localized in any one brain structure, trauma to one part of the nervous system can create initial memory loss, but some memory gradually returns even though the lesion or trauma seemed to have caused complete amnesia.

175. The answer is D. *(Kandel, 3/e, pp 999–1002).* Specific behavioral problems, such as shouting obscenities, messiness, or poor hygienic habits, that are often found in institutionalized psychiatric patients can be reduced and replaced with positive and constructive behavior through operant reinforcement by first precisely defining the behavior to be established, then finding an effective reinforcement (e.g., praise, attention, compliments, privileges, money, tokens, food), and finally training the staff to provide the appropriate reinforcement when the desired behavior is emitted by the patient. Punishment is not usually a part of operant reinforcement if one wishes to establish positive and constructive behavior.

176. The answer is A. *(Gatchel, 2/e, pp 85–93).* Repeated instances of noncontingent behavior and outcome can result in learned helplessness, with a person learning and expecting that most events are not controllable or will not be successful. A number of parallels have been drawn between learned helplessness and depression. Although both learned helplessness and depression are very complex phenomena, the characterizations of passive behavior, negative expectations ("I won't be able to do this"), hopelessness, and a feeling of having no control over life's events are present in both. Failing continuously because of one's lack of ability or skill is more apt to relate to depression, while failing because of one's feeling of lack of control over outcomes is more apt to lead to a feeling of helplessness.

177. The answer is C. *(Gatchel, 2/e, pp 116–118.)* Biofeedback and relaxation training have been used to modify the stress-induced components of hypertension. This results in a small but significant reduction in blood pressure—frequently about 15 mmHg systolic and 10 mmHg diastolic. Meditation and yoga have also been effective in lowering blood pressure. These modest declines in blood pressure have been demonstrated to be especially effective with the person who is at the stage of mild or even moderate hypertension. Weight reduction accomplished by changing one's eating behaviors will also reduce one's blood pressure, even when the salt intake is held constant. Contingency conditioning has not proved effective.

178. The answer is C. *(Kandel, 3/e, pp 997–1002.)* Timing is critical in both classical and operant conditioning. In classical conditioning, the conditional stimulus and unconditional stimulus must be presented closely, otherwise learning is poor or slow. In operant conditioning, the reinforcer must follow the desired response without delay, or only weak conditioning will occur. The person or animal must be able to discriminate between the two stimuli (stimuli discrimination) in classical conditioning in order for the second stimulus to be able to elicit the response. Extinction occurs in classical conditioning if the conditional stimulus is repeatedly presented without the unconditional stimulus. Likewise, if reinforcement is not given when the desired response occurs in operant conditioning, the probability of the response's occurring decreases until the response eventually ceases. Simultaneous stimuli presentation is relevant for classical conditioning but not necessary for operant conditioning. Classical conditioning is usually restricted to a specific reflex response (e.g., salivation) that is evoked by a specific stimulus (e.g., food). Operant conditioning involves any behavior that will tend to repeat itself if properly rewarded (reinforced). The learning of predictive relationships between stimuli and behaviors is important in both classical and operant conditioning. In classical conditioning, the person (animal) learns that a certain stimulus (food) predicts a subsequent stimulus (bell) or event. In operant conditioning, the person learns to predict the consequences by his or her behavior as the result of its being reinforced (rewarded).

179. The answer is E. *(Lerner, Psychology, pp 419–425.)* Social learning theory suggests that all the following are methods of attitude change: direct reinforcement—rewarding an expression of the desired attitude or behavior; extinction—denying the rewards that maintain the attitude that is to be changed; and modeling—watching someone else being rewarded for desired responses and punished for undesired ones. Desensitization is a technique for conditioning neutral or positive responses to previously fear-inducing stimuli. It, too, is based on social learning principles. Social learning theory is based primarily on considerations of nurture and has done very little to attempt to integrate considerations of nature (i.e., biologic factors).

180. The answer is C. *(Kandel, 3/e, pp 1001–1002.)* Systematic desensitization was developed by Joseph Wolpe in an effort to decrease neurotic anxiety or phobias that are learned and are usually precipitated by certain environmental situations, such as fear of heights or crowds. The patient is taught muscular relaxation; then, while using the relaxation to inhibit the anxiety, the patient is told to imagine a series of progressively more severe anxiety-provoking situations (e.g., climbing to the second step of a ladder, then the fourth step, and so on) until the anxiety-provoking situation of the highest (strongest) level can be brought to mind without the accompanying anxiety or fear. The anxiety-provoking situation is not brought to mind to be treated by any special form of psychotherapy but becomes paired with the anxiety-reducing relaxation. Most of these anxiety-provoking situations are situation-specific; however, the desensitization often generalizes to other real-life situations that may be potentially anxiety-provoking.

181. The answer is C. *(Sierles, pp 10–11.)* Prevention is still the best hope for controlling the HIV epidemic, and strategies dealing with the perception of health risk and leading to the change of high-risk behavior have proved most effective. While knowledge alone is insufficient to change behaviors that are so powerfully reinforced by pleasurable experiences, it can become an important factor when combined with other strategies of behavioral change, especially modifying how persons perceive the seriousness of the health risk, their vulnerability, and the benefits and personal costs of changing versus not changing one's behavior in the interests of health. The training of peers as endorsers of behavioral change has proved effective in the homosexual community, as has the implementation of needle-exchange programs among IV drug users. Strategies emphasizing disapproval, negative attitudes, fear, or rejection have not proved to be effective. Physicians can play a major role in the promotion of healthy behavioral change, as can social support from valued individuals and groups.

182. The answer is A. *(Schneiderman, pp 487–489.)* The migraine headache is associated with vascular dysfunction. The headache is typically preceded by intense constriction of the intra- and extracranial arteries in the temporal region. This is followed by a rebound dilation of the vasculature and then a sterile inflammation and edema of the arteries. Medication and psychotherapy are only marginally effective. By using biofeedback of finger skin temperature with the patient imagining a feeling of warmth in the fingers and hands, vasodilation is produced in peripheral blood vessels. The patient learns to control the dilation of peripheral blood vessels, which is also associated with constriction of cranial arteries. Patients taught to constrict their temporal arteries have also reported decreases in headache activity compared with controls. Similar results were demonstrated using EMG biofeedback with the frontalis muscle. Patients using such biofeedback technology have reported fewer and shorter headaches and less use of pain pills. This has not only been effective in the clinic but has been practiced at home without instrumentation. Subsequent research has also demonstrated the effectiveness of relaxation training in reducing general sympathetic tone. Systematic desensitization is also effective and augments the effect of relaxation so that the individual patient can identify and reduce specific stress responses.

183. The answer is C. *(Rosen, p 24.)* Social learning theory, developed by Bandura, suggests that through observation children acquire certain expectations and learned behavior with regard to smoking. Through media and models they can learn vicariously, for example, that smoking appears to relieve tension or anxiety. Also, when they observe a model appearing to enjoy the behavior, and without negative consequences, a condition of disinhibition results. The young person's learned expectation of negative consequences does not occur, and the expectation of negative consequences becomes weakened. This becomes an important factor in the ultimate decision regarding smoking.

184.   The answer is C. *(Rosen, pp 219–222.)* There is a wide range of intervention strategies and technologies, many of which are very successful (e.g., 50 to 70 percent), but the relapse rate is also high, especially during the first 6 to 9 months after the behavioral change program has terminated. This emphasizes the need to continue some strategy to sustain the behavior, as one might continue to prescribe a drug for hypertension or diabetes. While the behavioral technology for changing behavior is well developed, we are not so well informed about how to prepare and motivate people to decide to adopt risk reduction and health promotion regimens. Outstanding progress has been made on identifying and modifying risk factors and risk behavior, but we know much less about health promotion, since promoting health is far more complex than eliminating risk factors and risk behaviors. Lastly, a far greater percentage of people are able to successfully initiate, complete, and maintain risk-reducing behaviors if they do so on their own. This success appears to be related to self-direction, but little is known about how this occurs, just as medicine knows little about how certain illnesses or conditions abate without medical intervention.

185.   The answer is D. *(Rosen, pp 134–140.)* In general, there are three major interactive strategies used in attempting to change type A patterns of behavior: changing the environmental demands, changing the patient's responses to the environment (both behavioral and cognitive), and changing the physiologic concomitants of type A behaviors. Examples of counteracting certain environmental demands or triggers include limiting time spent in the environment, rescheduling deadlines, or avoiding interruptions. Changing one's response is best accomplished by learning to observe one's own type A behaviors (e.g., anger or hostility) and then contracting with oneself to alter those behaviors by practicing new behaviors, coping styles, or reactions. Progressive relaxation, biofeedback, and exercising are effective methods of reducing many of the physiologic responses to stress and anxiety. Attempting to change the expectations of a social group or society is very difficult, especially if the changes are to be directed at one's own personal needs.

186.   The answer is D. *(Rosen, pp 26–30.)* The modeling of parents, teachers, and "significant others" has been found to play a major role in influencing a person to smoke. Peer pressure is also a major influence, especially in adolescence. Cigarette advertising, which may use celebrity models and link smoking to such attractions as sports, sex, and prestige, impresses youth with the pleasurable, grown-up, and no-risk aspects of smoking. Social inoculation is a process whereby persons are inoculated with arguments and behavioral skills to reinforce the effects of positive modeling, the social skills to counteract peer pressure to smoke, and various content analyses of the techniques used by advertisers to persuade youth to smoke. Experimentation is a common characteristic of adolescence and smoking is one of the most frequent behavioral trials.

187. The answer is D. *(Isselbacher, 13/e, pp 446–452.)* Empirical studies have revealed a number of changes in eating habits that will significantly discourage the tendency to eat more food than is required by the body. Nutritional experts recommend that we eat more slowly, serve ourselves smaller portions, wait at least 20 min after we have eaten our first serving before taking a second serving, restrict all our eating to one or two places in the home, do not watch television or read while we are eating, and let family and friends know that we are trying to cut down on food intake. In addition we should go grocery shopping only after we have eaten a satisfying meal, not leave food out where we repeatedly see it and can easily reach it many times a day, try to spend less time in the kitchen, get someone else in the family to clear the plates and put away the leftovers, and keep a detailed log or diary of all food intake. Such activities will help to disrupt previously learned, but inappropriate, eating behaviors and establish appropriate environmental conditions and eating behaviors.

188. The answer is E. *(Last, 13/e, pp 1094–1096.)* Physicians have to learn a set of specific educational skills in order to help their patients make significant and lasting changes in their health-related behavior. Several empirical studies have suggested strategies that can be used for improving the effectiveness of health services. Among other strategies, the physician should provide continuity of personalized medical care, discover and respond to the patient's expectations in an individualized manner, simplify the health regimen as much as possible, and provide health knowledge that is necessary to support the recommended behavior and is action-oriented. The physician should also make the health behaviors and motives important to the patient and family, maximize the rewards for the prescribed health-related behavior, minimize the cost and inconveniences, try working slowly into regimens that are unpleasant, and instill a sense of personal responsibility in the patient for his or her own health maintenance.

189. The answer is D. *(Feuerstein, pp 438–445.)* Pain and pain-related behavior can be influenced by the environment via basic learning mechanisms. This concept has made a major contribution to the understanding and management of chronic pain. It recognizes that the pain behavior itself (the overt actions and reactions of the person) is significant in its own right and not necessarily attributed to some underlying anxiety or conflict. Also, it emphasizes operational measurement and observation of the pain behavior itself (e.g., moaning, inactivity, use of medications), not the pain or inferred concepts as to why the person is feeling or reacting to pain. Using these concepts, the pain behavior can be conditioned as separate from the pain itself. Operant conditioning mechanisms are involved as the pain behavior is affected by such environmental consequences as reward (positive) or punishment (negative) factors, which act as reinforcers.

190. The answer is E. *(Feuerstein, pp 438–445.)* The environment can influence pain-related behavior via learning mechanisms, principally operant conditioning, respondent or classical conditioning, and modeling or observational learning. This is referred to as the *learning mechanisms hypothesis.* Certain rewards or secondary gains from the environment (e.g., reduced work or increased attention) are involved in operant behavior mechanisms of reward and reinforcement. The respondent conditioning mechanism involves a specific antecedent; for example, a person may link increased lumbar pain with sleep time so that the pain and preparing for sleep become associated, with the result of anticipatory anxiety and increased pain at bed time. A similar anticipatory or avoidance behavior can maintain such behaviors as limping or decreased activity. Observational learning (or vicarious learning, or modeling) refers to learned reactions to pain as observed in parents, peers, and family or through role expectation. A parent who consistently avoids work when ill can be a model for a child who learns to avoid school or responsibility.

191. The answer is A. *(Ader, 2/e, pp 638–640.)* The functional relationship between the nervous system and the immune system has been demonstrated by the ability to condition alterations of immune responses. The evidence is compelling and is based on such findings as the ability to condition immune suppression or enhancement of antibody- and cell-mediated immune responses, the ability to extinguish such conditioned responses, the development of tolerance to an immunomodulating agent, and the immunologic effects of stress that have been conditioned. Conditioning effects have also been observed using antigens as unconditioned stimuli. Thus far, studies have been unable to demonstrate conditioned compensatory responses in the immune system, but there have been some inferences of compensatory mechanisms.

192–195. The answers are 192-E, 193-D, 194-C, 195-B. *(Gatchel, 2/e, pp 217–229.)* Classical conditioning is a basic form of learning. It was first described by Ivan Pavlov working on the conditioned reflex. He was able to take an autonomic reflex (e.g., salivation to food) which was thought to be unconditioned and demonstrated that it could be conditioned to respond to a new stimulus (e.g., a bell) if the new stimulus was presented along with or prior to the unconditioned stimulus (food). After a number of such presentations the new stimulus (bell) would elicit the autonomic unconditioned response. The autonomic response had, in effect, learned to respond to the new stimulus (i.e., a learned association or connection between the two stimuli had occurred). Pavlov called this learned association *stimulus substitution.*

Operant conditioning, sometimes called *instrumental conditioning*, was formulated by Edward Thorndike and later developed by B. F. Skinner. In operant conditioning a new behavioral response is learned, as compared with classical conditioning in which a new stimulus is conditioned (learned) to elicit the same response or behavior. In operant conditioning reinforcement becomes the key stimulus that increases the likelihood that the desired behavior will be repeated or strengthened.

Systematic desensitization is a behavioral technique developed on basic principles of classical conditioning. Joseph Wolpe developed it as a means of alleviating anxiety. Deep muscle relaxation is paired with a series of imagined scenes that depict situations or objects that are associated with anxiety and thus produce anxiety. The scenes or situations are graded into a hierarchy and the pairing with relaxation proceeds from the most simple to the most severe scenes. The patient thus learns to tolerate more and more severe or difficult scenes and becomes desensitized as the relaxation acts to inhibit the anxiety response. The behavioral technique has been especially effective with phobias, insomnia, and stress-related disorders.

Shaping is a reinforcement and learning process wherein a series of successive responses that approximate the desired response are reinforced until the desired response is learned. It is basically an operant conditioning procedure and was originally developed using the bar-pressing response of rats as the act to be learned. The rat was positively reinforced for each of the closer and closer approximations, such as approaching the bar, rising upon hind legs, putting front paws on the bar (lever), and pressing the bar. This is also known as the successive approximation shaping procedure. After the desired behavior has been learned, the experimenter can then introduce different reinforcement schedules to maintain the learned behavior. A discriminative stimulus can also be introduced, such as pressing the bar only when a certain light is on, so that the animal will learn not to press the bar except when the light is on. The shaping technique has been used to train circus and other animals to perform complicated acts used in most zoo and marine animal shows. The process of shaping is considered to be prominent, although greatly modified, in many social and cultural learning situations of everyday life.

Contact desensitization is a variation of systematic desensitization that combines modeling and guided participation procedures. In a fearful person, the therapist (or teacher) models the appropriate behavior and then guides the fearful person through each step of a hierarchy. Contact desensitization has been very effective in the treatment of phobias, such as the fear of snakes. The therapist would model appropriate behaviors, such as approaching the snake, touching the snake, and progressively allowing the snake to crawl around the therapist's arms and shoulders. The fearful person is then encouraged to perform each of these behaviors, beginning with the lowest behavioral task in the hierarchy. With the assistance of the therapist, each behavioral task is repeated until the fear and anxiety associated with the snake are extinguished. This method differs from systematic desensitization in that while a hierarchy is used, relaxation training is not. The procedure is based on extinction rather than depending on relaxation to inhibit the anxiety.

196–197. The answers are 196-E, 197-C. *(Sierles, pp 74–76.)* The woman who became nauseous prior to chemotherapy demonstrates a case of classical conditioning as developed by Pavlov. In his famous experiment, he gave meat powder to a dog and noted the unconditioned response (UCR) of salivation. He then paired the meat powder with a bell (unconditioned stimulus) and eventually was able to make the dog salivate at the sound of the bell (conditioned response) alone. A similar classical conditioning occurs when a patient associates some aspect of the oncology clinic (e.g., the room, smell, sight of the intravenous infusion bottle) with the nausea previously experienced during the intravenous process itself. Thus, the mere sight or smell of one or more components of the experience can produce the conditioned response of nausea and vomiting. A similar type of conditioning (fear or anxiety) can occur in a child at the sight of a white coat after having experienced a shot or other painful procedure, or in an adult whose blood pressure can increase at the prospect of having blood pressure measured for hypertension.

The decline in responsiveness or reaction to the repeated presentation of a stimulus is known as *habituation*. Thus, a medical student may feel very queasy in the first few days or weeks in the anatomy laboratory, or when exposed to blood in surgery, or in dealing with an intoxicated or violent patient in the emergency room, but after multiple exposures, habituation takes place and the student becomes more comfortable in that setting. Habituation can also be a part of an effective therapeutic process in patients with certain phobias, fears, troubling thoughts, or obsessive-compulsive behaviors. When presented with anxiety-producing stimuli of various intensities over time, these patients may become habituated to the stimuli.

In negative reinforcement, the unpleasant stimulus is removed, contingent on a desired response.

Modeling is the presentation of another person (usually of high status or recognized experience) as a model of desired behavior.

Instrumental (operant) conditioning is a mechanism for increasing the probability of a response by introducing a reward or reinforcement. B. F. Skinner pioneered the study of behavior that anticipates a reward or reinforcement. This reinforcement can be either positive or negative.

198–199. The answers are 198-C, 199-A. *(Sierles, pp 77–78.)* The female patient is engaged in a fixed-interval schedule of reinforcement. While this may not be a desirable procedure for the patient's health, she has adopted it as a way of coping with a requirement. By establishing a fixed-interval checkup, the physician may have unwittingly allowed the patient too many opportunities to avoid adherence to the dietary component of the program. A variable-interval schedule or some other means of monitoring the adherence and the weight could have produced a better result. An on-call checkup would be an example of a variable-interval schedule. Behavior established with a variable-interval schedule will also be sustained for a longer period of time and is less easily extinguished.

Stimulus control is an attempt to limit or exclude certain stimuli or cues that tend to trigger certain behaviors. Studies of eating behavior have found that many persons are stimulated to eat by cues (e.g., the presence of food, a comfortable environment, or a commercial interlude on television), resulting in the consumption of excess calories that maintain or increase their obesity. By attempting to identify and eliminate such environmental cues (stimulus control), one can reduce or eliminate unwanted behaviors. Stimulus control is also effective in programs for cessation of smoking. The goal is to reduce or eliminate specific stressful situations (e.g., interpersonal encounters) or environments (e.g., the smoking section in a restaurant) that may serve as a cue to reach for and to smoke a cigarette.

In desensitization, one is attempting to reduce the reaction to a stimulus to which the patient has become oversensitized. This is usually related to a phobia or anxiety reaction. An effective therapeutic procedure would be to identify a hierarchy of fear responses and work to desensitize the patient's responses from the least to the most severe.

A variable-ratio reinforcement is best illustrated by a slot machine player, who may be rewarded after 6 lever pulls, again after only 3 pulls, but next after 20 pulls. The person is motivated to continue to play and at an increased number of pulls. A variable-ratio schedule is most resistant to extinction.

200–201. The answers are 200-B, 201-E. *(Sierles, pp 76–79.)* The smoker is being exposed to an aversive stimulus. The physiologic and psychological trauma is so severe and so aversive that the patient may choose to avoid smoking in the future. This can also be regarded as a form of punishment. In positive punishment, an unpleasant stimulus is applied, such as spanking or other acts that produce pain; in negative punishment, a positive reinforcer is removed (e.g., withdrawing use of the family car or other privileges). While punishment is not as effective in changing behavior as other more positive reinforcers, it can be effective, at least in dangerous situations and for the short term. Punishment during a longer period can produce resentment, it does not demonstrate positive alternative behaviors, and with certain persons (e.g., a child or adult who is seeking attention) it can become a substitute for positive reinforcement (i.e., the attention gained during spanking can sometimes outweigh the pain).

Systematic desensitization can reduce anxiety in a situation by identifying a hierarchy of situations that produce anxiety from low to high. For example, the bridge designer can be taught progressive muscle relaxation until he is as relaxed as possible, at which point he will begin by driving across the shortest or least anxiety-producing bridge (in vivo exposure). As he successfully experiences crossing the lowest anxiety-producing bridge, he can proceed up the hierarchy of bridges until he masters crossing the most anxiety-producing bridge. This process of systematic desensitization can also be used cognitively if, after identifying the hierarchy, he can practice muscle relaxation, fantasize about crossing the lowest bridge without becoming anxious, and then proceed up the hierarchy. This principle can also be used to treat anxiety over such situations as going to the dentist or entering a crowded room, or a number of anxiety phobias. The muscle relaxation involves an important principle of reciprocal inhibition—a person cannot be relaxed and anxious simultaneously.

202–205. The answers are 202-E, 203-A, 204-B, 205-C. *(Gatchel, 2/e, pp 227–234.)* From studying a mnemonist and various yogi experts who could control their heart rates, skin temperatures, and other physiologic processes, it was documented that an average person can learn to accomplish the same control by using certain visual or auditory feedback cues. We learn skills and everyday behaviors by using the basic learning principle that we can learn and improve performance by receiving feedback about our response and then making appropriate adjustments. Learning to drive a car, throw a baseball, or perform a venipuncture requires continuous feedback. By providing visual or auditory feedback (biofeedback) of physiologic responses, we can also learn to control voluntarily such physiologic functions. Pioneering experiments by Neal Miller in the late 1950s and early 1960s with animals were extended to demonstrate human subjects' ability to learn to control many responses that were assumed to be "involuntary responses," such as blood pressure, heart rate, activity of the sweat glands, skin temperature, neuromuscular activity, and various brain rhythms. The clinical application of the behavioral technology of biofeedback continues to be explored and effectively applied to certain disorders, such as hypertension, Raynaud's disease, migraine headache, asthma, gastrointestinal disorders, dyskinesias, epileptic seizures, cardiac arrhythmias, anxiety, headache from muscle contraction, and muscular pain.

Contingency management is an attempt to control or manage the contingency between reinforcement (reward) and certain behavior (e.g., pressing a bar) in order to increase the frequency of that behavior. It involves systematically controlling the consequences with appropriate reinforcement. This method is used extensively in everyday activities to encourage or discourage certain behaviors in children, patients, or others with whom we relate. As an example, token economy programs, which give tokens as exchangeable awards, have proved to be very effective in treatment and rehabilitation, especially when the goal is to decrease undesirable behavior, psychotic talk, or the bizarre patterns of behavior of schizophrenics. The contingency management methods are also very effective in increasing the frequency of socially adaptive behaviors, responsibility, and self-reliance.

Cognitive restructuring is a therapeutic technique based on the fundamental discovery by Albert Ellis (1962) that cognitions and faulty or irrational patterns of thinking can produce emotions and other psychological disorders, such as anxiety. By changing the internal or covert sentences that people say to themselves, they can reduce or eliminate negative emotional responses. This became known as cognitive restructuring, and while it may sound deceptively simple, it has added further confirmation to earlier studies showing that not only do attitudes affect behavior, changing behavior also affects attitudes. By integrating the biobehavioral perspective, we can demonstrate how specific thoughts or verbalizations to oneself can give rise to the psychological and physiologic aspects of anxiety. By identifying and modifying (restructuring) these negative verbalizations to oneself and replacing them with more positive statements to oneself, anxiety can be reduced. Similar to systematic desensitization, cognitive restructuring has demonstrated in controlled experiments that it is highly effective in reducing anxiety. Systematic desensitization is more effective with certain phobias, and cognitive restructuring is more effective with multiple fears in interpersonal situations.

Thought-stopping is a variation of restructuring. The client concentrates on specific anxiety-producing thoughts, which are then interrupted by a sudden shock statement "stop" by the therapist. After several interruptions, the locus of control is then shifted to the client by the client's learning to emit a subvocal "stop" at any time he or she begins to engage in the self-defeating rumination. In another technique, the client snaps a rubber band worn on his or her wrist when such ruminations occur. Even though this has a slight punishing effect, it does serve to provide an impressive "stop" signal and interrupts the destructive thinking. The thought-stopping procedures are especially effective with clients who have difficulty controlling distressing obsessional thoughts. The techniques of cognitive restructuring mentioned above can be effective in helping patients cope with psychological stressors that are linked to the precipitation exacerbation of physical symptoms. Again, what appears to be deceptively simple and superficial actually works and is based on more recent knowledge in neuroscience and behavioral science than are the traditional psychotherapeutic principles.

There has been much renewed interest in techniques of self-control and self-management for controlling problem behaviors. Some of the more successful techniques have been developed by working with patients attempting to control obesity but can also be applied to smoking, stress, tension, and other problems. Such techniques involve identifying significant rewards and punishments that can be used by patients to reinforce the behavior they are attempting to monitor and control. For example, in the control of obesity there is self-monitoring of daily weight, calories, and exercise; self-reward with extra money, purchases, or privileges; and self-punishment with fines and denial of special privileges or favored activity. Self-monitoring and self-reward are more effective reinforcers than is punishment. Social support is also an effective reinforcement for self-control.

Life-Span Development

DIRECTIONS: Each question below contains five suggested responses. Select the **one best** response to each question.

206. Erik Erikson views the stage of young adulthood as being best described by a crisis of

(A) trust versus mistrust
(B) intimacy versus isolation
(C) identity versus role confusion
(D) initiative versus guilt
(E) autonomy versus dependence

207. The environmental factor with the most underused potential for developing cognitive and interpersonal competence in children is the

(A) school
(B) family setting
(C) community mental health center
(D) health care system
(E) child welfare agency

208. According to current research, a daughter is most likely to have traditional vocational aspirations if she has a

(A) nonworking mother
(B) working mother
(C) mother in a traditionally masculine occupation
(D) working father
(E) father with high occupational status

209. Sequential studies of human development suggest that the growth of intelligence may continue through

(A) late adolescence
(B) early adulthood
(C) middle adulthood
(D) late adulthood
(E) old age

210. The leading nutritional problem among senior citizens in the Unites States is

(A) vitamin deficiencies
(B) fiber deficiency
(C) malnutrition
(D) undernutrition
(E) obesity

211. A prominent "embracing" response that can be elicited in a newborn infant by a sudden change in the head position is called the

(A) sign of Babinski
(B) startle (Moro's) reflex
(C) convulsive reflex
(D) infant carry response
(E) primate hug

212. Erik Erikson's theory of the life cycle and growth of the ego is reflected in which of the following statements?

(A) Sexual drive is crucial in determining the development of a sense of identity
(B) Ego maturation is genetically predetermined; cultural influences are of minor importance
(C) There are eight stages characterized by crises whose satisfactory resolution is essential to the development of a healthy sense of identity
(D) The phases of development are characterized in turn by aggressive, affiliative, achievement, nurturance, and power motives
(E) People are burdened with too many ego functions; society would benefit from stricter and more economic processes of socialization

213. The most rapidly increasing rate of mortality is found in

(A) infancy
(B) childhood
(C) adolescence
(D) middle age
(E) old age

214. The complex of symptoms characteristic of children who are deprived of their mother or of a mother substitute during infancy and often extending into the first years of life is known as

(A) stranger anxiety
(B) anxiety neurosis
(C) autism
(D) childhood schizophrenia
(E) anaclitic depression

215. Which of the following statements about the development of moral standards during childhood is true?

(A) Only at puberty do a child's moral standards become independent of external rewards and punishments

(B) The development of guilt as a reaction to transgressions is fostered by parental warmth

(C) Children of 11 or 12 years of age are more likely to make inflexible, absolute moral judgments than those 7 or 8 years of age

(D) Older children are more likely than younger children to judge behavior as right or wrong in terms of its reinforcement outcomes

(E) The development of moral reasoning is independent of general intellectual maturation

216. The most common presenting feature of Alzheimer's disease is

(A) change in personality

(B) loss of memory

(C) difficulty in learning new information

(D) impairment of orientation to time

(E) loss of intellectual skills

217. Language development in childhood is characterized by which of the following?

(A) Infants 15 to 20 weeks of age use different patterns of vocalization to identify discomforts such as hunger, fright, and pain

(B) Most children master all consonant sounds by the age of 3 to $3\frac{1}{2}$ years

(C) The first words spoken are usually verbs

(D) Vowels emerge in hierarchical order between ages $3\frac{1}{2}$ and 7 years

(E) None of the above

218. Significant changes in physiologic and cognitive functioning develop with age. Studies of aging show that

(A) intraindividual variability is decreased with aging

(B) interindividual variability is decreased with aging

(C) there is more age-related decline found in longitudinal methods than in cross-sectional methods

(D) life-style and experiences play a major role in retention of various cognitive functions

(E) sustained attention is reduced considerably by age 80

219. True statements concerning aging include which of the following?

(A) Twenty percent of aged persons live in long-stay institutions (nursing homes, mental hospitals, homes for the aged)

(B) The majority of old people feel bad most of the time

(C) Aged drivers have more accidents per person than drivers under age 65

(D) All five senses tend to decline in old age

(E) Personality traits become unstable in the elderly

DIRECTIONS: Each numbered question or incomplete statement below is NEGATIVELY phrased. Select the **one best** lettered response.

220. All the following statements about aging are true EXCEPT

(A) the maximal life span has increased in populations over the past 20 years
(B) the risk of death increases exponentially with time
(C) life expectancy would increase only 20 years if heart disease and cancer were eliminated
(D) the biomedical model is becoming increasingly inapplicable in accounting for death in the elderly
(E) the $\dot{V}_{O_{2max}}$ can be used as an integrated measure of the functional limits of the whole body

221. Educational stimulation of disadvantaged children results in a subsequent improvement in cognitive and academic performance when stimulation includes all the following EXCEPT

(A) daily rather than occasional activity
(B) maintenance for an extensive period of time
(C) very early institution of aid
(D) a focus on cognitive, language, and number skills
(E) attempts to separate these children from the influence of their family

222. Compared with pregnant women aged 20 to 25, pregnant adolescents are more apt to have all the following EXCEPT

(A) infants of lower birth weight
(B) inadequate prenatal care
(C) higher rates of infant mortality
(D) similar rates of birth defects and mental retardation
(E) higher degree of poverty

223. All the following research findings on adult development are true EXCEPT that

(A) significant developmental changes continue to occur throughout adulthood
(B) as people age, there is an increasing range of differences between individuals
(C) changes in adulthood occur in all areas of development (cognitive, physical, and social-personal)
(D) adult cognitive changes may show quantitative reduction on an ability test, but a qualitative acquisition of a different form of intelligence
(E) just as is the case in childhood and adolescence, there are predominant and universal developmental stages in adulthood

224. In comparing health behaviors of younger and older people, older people report all the following EXCEPT

(A) more symptoms
(B) less positive health status
(C) more vulnerability to health threats
(D) decline in regular physical activity
(E) improvement of eating habits

225. Recent studies concerned with alcohol use and abuse in adolescence have found all the following to be true EXCEPT that

(A) alcohol is the most widely used drug by youth between the ages of 12 and 17
(B) adolescent problem drinkers are less likely to use illicit drugs than are nondrinkers
(C) heavy drinking during adolescence is typically accompanied by other antisocial behaviors
(D) the most frequent cause of death and disability among youth today is traffic accidents, many of which are directly related to alcohol
(E) adolescent problem drinkers are more tolerant of deviance

226. In René Spitz's classic study of sensory deprivation, he found all the following to be true EXCEPT that

(A) social interaction with other humans is essential in infant development
(B) in the first 4 months, infants in the foundling home (having less contact with other people) scored better on several developmental indices than those in the nursing home (where mothers visited)
(C) by 1 year, the foundling home infants had fallen far below those in the nursing home on developmental indices
(D) after 2 or 3 years, most infants in the foundling home could not walk or talk
(E) children in the nursing home had a higher incidence of infection than those in the foundling home because of the many social contacts

227. Stages in the child's normal development of speech are characterized by all the following statements EXCEPT that

(A) between 1 and 6 months, infants invent new noises and experiment with them
(B) infants 4 to 5 months old will repeat sounds they hear
(C) infants between 12 and 18 months will intentionally use a word appropriate to the situation
(D) between 24 and 36 months, infants use 200 to 300 words in phrases and two-word sentences
(E) by 48 months of age, the child should have a vocabulary of about 1500 words

228. All the following factors are included in gender identity EXCEPT

(A) gender role behavior
(B) parental and cultural attitudes
(C) external genitalia
(D) sexual behavior
(E) genetic influence

229. Research findings on early gender-role identification and behaviors show that all the following statements are true EXCEPT

(A) gender-related differences in play behavior are evident as early as 13 months
(B) males are generally more aggressive in their play and problem-solving activities than are females
(C) children who experience gender reassignment after the age of 2 are considered to be high-risk candidates for psychological disorders
(D) children between 3 and 4 years of age are able to make gender-appropriate choices according to Western stereotypes
(E) females 3 to 5 years old appear to be more concerned about gender-appropriate play activities than are males of a similar age

230. In comparing overweight adolescent boys and girls, girls are more apt to experience all the following EXCEPT

(A) parental pressure to restrict food intake
(B) inclination to eat in response to negative and positive moods
(C) blame by their parents for their weight status
(D) presence of other people as a signal for eating
(E) inclination to take more drastic measures to control their weight

231. The phenomenon of parent-infant bonding proposed by Kennell and Klaus produces all the following EXCEPT

(A) enhancement of infant's language development
(B) enhancement of infant's cognitive development
(C) increase in parental touching and fondling
(D) decrease in amount of crying done by infant
(E) increase in unwarranted maternal concern

232. Which of the following factors is LEAST powerful in the development of a child's identification with a parent?

(A) Perception of physical and behavioral similarities
(B) Communication from others concerning similarities
(C) Imitation of parental mannerisms
(D) Attractiveness of the parent
(E) Obedience to parental authority

233. Intelligence and cognitive development during adolescence are usually characterized by each of the following EXCEPT

(A) the emergence of hypothetico-deductive reasoning
(B) attitudes and reasoning that tend to be egocentric
(C) a growing capacity for probabilistic thinking
(D) a type of reasoning that subordinates reality to possibility
(E) less attention to and ability to infer what others are thinking and feeling

234. Perinatal gonadal hormones have a developmental impact on all the following EXCEPT

(A) sex-linked neural differentiation
(B) sexuality in adulthood
(C) neural morphology
(D) the permanent organization of parts of the nervous system
(E) hermaphroditism in genetic males

235. Cognitive skills of early childhood show all the following patterns EXCEPT

(A) at 18 months, a child begins to follow simple one-part directions, begins many questions with "what," imitates people in his or her environment, and infers causes from observing effects

(B) at 2 years, the child begins to learn about time sequences, matches simple shapes and sizes, attempts new solutions to old problems, and may arrange several words in grammatically incorrect sentences

(C) at 3 years, the child asks many "why" questions, talks in sentences using four or more words, can give his first and last name, and may talk about his fears

(D) at 4 years, the child may begin many questions with "how," knows the days of the week, can identify coins correctly, and can follow a three-step direction in proper order

(E) at 5 years, the child asks the meaning of words, talks more, and is more externally focused

236. Biologic changes in the adolescent years include all the following EXCEPT

(A) a growth spurt for girls with peak velocity at 14 years of age

(B) menarche at any time between 10 and $16\frac{1}{2}$ years of age; the average now is just over 12 years of age

(C) a growth spurt for boys with peak velocity about 2 years later than girls

(D) growth of testes beginning as early as age $9\frac{1}{2}$ or as late as age $13\frac{1}{2}$ and ending at any time between ages $13\frac{1}{2}$ and 17 years

(E) a historical rate of decreased age of menarche of about 4 months each decade

237. Concepts of death and pain at various stages of child development include all the following EXCEPT

(A) between birth and 2 years of age, separation is more apt to be experienced as synonymous with death

(B) children 3 and 4 years of age believe that a toy feels pain when it is broken

(C) children 5 to 6 years old fantasize that the dead person continues to experience emotion and biologic function in the grave

(D) children 7 to 9 years of age realize the inevitability of death for all living things, no longer feel responsible for the death of others, and yet feel that death can be avoided

(E) at 10 to 12 years of age children see death as the result of aggression or trauma and can accept the concept of nonexistence

DIRECTIONS: Each group of questions below consists of lettered headings followed by a set of numbered items. For each numbered item select the **one** lettered heading with which it is **most** closely associated. Each lettered heading may be used **once, more than once, or not at all**.

Questions 238–241

For each description of a child's behavior below, select the age with which it is most closely associated as part of the growth and development sequence.

- (A) 18 months
- (B) 2 years
- (C) 3 years
- (D) 4 years
- (E) 5 years

238. Cuts around pictures with scissors; buttons a small button; can copy a square

239. Can drink from a cup without much spilling; turns several pages of a book together; builds a tower of four or five blocks

240. Can copy a circle; can wash and dry hands; can brush teeth—but not adequately; begins to use blunt scissors

241. Can turn doorknobs that can be reached; can drink from small cup using one hand; builds a tower of six or seven blocks

Questions 242–244

Match each view of illness with the developmental age at which it is characteristic.

- (A) Preschool age
- (B) Elementary school age
- (C) High school age
- (D) Adult
- (E) Elderly

242. Person views self as immortal or immune to external agents (e.g., germs)

243. Person regards illness as a consequence of "bad" behavior

244. Person fears loss of control

Life-Span Development
Answers

206. The answer is B. *(Lerner, Psychology, pp 334–343.)* Erik Erikson's stage theory of psychosocial development provides descriptions of personality development that are consistent with a life-span perspective. It has served as a major basis for research on human development. Erikson viewed the individual as having to develop the capacities (the ego functions) to meet the expectations of society. At each of the eight stages of psychosocial development there is an accompanying "ego crisis." These stages are trust versus mistrust (birth to $1\frac{1}{2}$ years), autonomy versus shame or doubt ($1\frac{1}{2}$ to 3 years), initiative versus guilt (3 to 6 years), industry versus inferiority (6 years to puberty), identity versus role confusion (adolescence), intimacy versus isolation (young adulthood), generativity versus stagnation (adulthood), and integrity versus despair (maturity). During intimacy versus isolation in the stage of young adulthood, there is psychosocial pressure for a person to form a close, stable interpersonal relationship. Thus, to the extent that one can attain an unconditional interchange and relationship, one will feel a sense of intimacy in feelings, ideas, and goals. If one cannot share and be shared, then one will feel a sense of isolation.

207. The answer is A. *(Hamburg, pp 81–89).* Cognitive and interpersonal competence are valued by society and incompetence can predispose to the development of psychopathology. Prevention and treatment through environmental factors have been shown to be effective in assisting the development of cognitive and interpersonal competence. The school environment is considered to have the most potential as a focus for intervention, but it is also the most underused resource at present. Schools can be effective as a buffer against negative or destructive environments, especially if they emphasize expectations of high achievement, provide positive feedback, allow children to assume responsibility within the school system, provide adequate discipline, and avoid physical punishment in dealing with learning or behavioral problems.

Intervention in discordant family settings, some types of institutionalization, community mental health centers, and the health care system can achieve limited success, but they are generally costly, isolated, and without the potential for multidisciplinary efforts.

208. The answer is A. *(Lerner, Psychology, pp 388–391.)* When females develop within a family in which their mother is employed, they have less stereotyped views of female roles than do daughters of nonworking mothers, have a broader definition of female roles, and are more likely to emulate their mothers. It is hypothesized that homes with working mothers have different family interactions than do homes with nonworking mothers. The modeling influence for working and the development of achievement orientations appear to be major factors in developing nontraditional vocational aspirations. Also, fathers of high occupational status are more apt to promote nontraditional vocational achievement in their daughters. Interaction in such family settings may promote the development of vocational role orientations and behaviors that are nontraditional. In contrast, the daughter of a nonworking mother will be more influenced by the traditional model of the nonworking mother and will develop achievement orientations more consistent with the traditional female roles.

209. The answer is E. *(Lerner, Psychology, pp 229–232.)* Studies of intelligence suggest that a person's IQ score is somewhat variable in the early years, becomes increasingly stable through middle adolescence, and at about age 18 reaches a maximum score that is maintained for some time. Early cross-sectional studies indicated a decrease in IQ scores from middle adolescence into adulthood, but data from later longitudinal research indicated more stability or actual increases in scores. In 1956, Schaie began to study 500 people ranging in age from 21 to 70. When the data were analyzed cross-sectionally, the adolescent-to-adulthood decline typically seen in such studies was observed, but when the data were looked at longitudinally within each of the birth cohort groups in their sequential design, a decline on only one of the four measures (visual-motor flexibility) of intelligence was found. Knowledge attained through education and socialization (e.g., verbal comprehension, number skills) and the ability to organize and process visual information resulted in a systematic increase in scores for all age groups. Clearly, the course of intellectual change from adolescence onward is not just an age-related phenomenon. One may expect that many of the levels and types of ability present in adolescence will be maintained or enhanced in the adult and aged years, in large part depending on such factors as education, experiences, and cognitive activities.

210. The answer is E. *(Sierles, p 167.)* Obesity is the leading nutritional problem of older persons in the United States. It affects one in five senior citizens and is reported to be increasing. Overnutrition (too many calories), lack of exercise, high-fat diet, and lack of balanced diet are the major contributing factors, with overnutrition and lack of exercise sharing major responsibility. Vitamin deficiency, fiber deficiency, and undernutrition (often due to poor dentition, poverty, or living alone) are contributing factors to obesity, but of lesser influence. The assessment of life-style and nutrition (including eating habits) is especially important in all interviews of the elderly because the cumulative effects of life-style factors such as smoking, lack of exercise, obesity, and alcoholism take their toll as patients age.

211. The answer is B. *(Schuster, 3/e, pp 104–105.)* Moro's reflex, known as the startle reflex, is significant in evaluating an infant's neurologic status. It is an innate response to unexpected changes in head position, or sometimes to any surprising event. The reflex involves extension of the arms laterally, extension of the fingers, and then return of hands to midline as if grasping or embracing someone. Developmentally, this reflex begins to disappear at 3 to 4 months and is usually gone by 6 months of age. It is believed that the disappearance of Moro's reflex coincides with functional maturation of the neocortex. Presumably, the cortex inhibits brainstem centers that mediate such early reflex responses.

212. The answer is C. *(Lerner, Encyclopedia, pp 321–323.)* Erik Erikson's theory of ego development defines eight "crises" during the life cycle. Each crisis is critical to the development of a sense of personal identity. Although these crises are partly related to the five stages of psychosexual development delineated by classic psychoanalysis, Erikson tends to give greater emphasis to the growth of ego functions as independent of libidinal drive and more related to psychosocial than psychosexual development. As such, they are related to adaptive demands placed on the individual by society and involve a life-span perspective. The eight crises are basic trust versus basic mistrust, autonomy versus shame and doubt, initiative versus guilty functioning, industry versus inferiority, identity versus role confusion, intimacy versus isolation, generativity versus stagnation, and integrity versus despair.

213. The answer is C. *(Hamburg, pp 130–131.)* In general, the mortality for adolescence is relatively low. However, adolescence is the only age period in which the mortality is actually rising. The potential loss is even greater for adolescents and for society when one calculates the years of life lost and loss of potential productivity over the life span. Among males, the leading cause of deaths is accidents, especially motor vehicle accidents.

214. The answer is E. *(Kaplan, 7/e, pp 43, 163–164.)* Anaclitic depression refers to the complex of symptoms exhibited by young children who are deprived of their mother or of a mother surrogate during the first few years of life. This reaction is made up of a number of stages. On first being separated from its caretaker, an infant will protest vigorously. If the caretaking figure is not restored to the infant, the infant enters what is known as the phase of despair and ceases protesting. This phase can be followed by a refusal to eat, which sometimes is fatal, or by a phase of detachment in which the infant withdraws from any interaction and engages in various forms of self-stimulation.

215. The answer is B. *(Schuster, 3/e, pp 337–345.)* While the cognitive development the child undergoes brings about a great awareness of moral values and standards, orientation to abiding by them depends on other factors, primarily identification with the parents and the experiencing of guilt for violation of guidelines. The development of conscience can be seen in internal reactions to transgressions in the form of guilt or by the child's taking up of standards that the child feels personally responsible for maintaining. A number of studies indicate that conscience development is fostered by the presence of parental love and warmth of a degree adequate for positive identification and modeling. Such positive identification and modeling more readily occur if the parents' own conscience and moral standards are mature and reasonable rather than either deficient or overly strict, harsh, and inflexible.

216. The answer is B. *(Hazzard, 3/e, pp 1036–1037.)* Alzheimer's disease is a progressive, disabling, degenerative disease and the most common cause of dementia in the elderly. The most common presenting feature of Alzheimer's disease is loss of memory. It is also usually accompanied by a gradual decline in intellectual function and impairment of orientation to time and place, judgment, problem solving, language, perception, and learning. Personality change often involves alteration or accentuation of premorbid traits, delusions, apathy, or depression.

217. The answer is A. *(Schuster, 3/e, pp 261–262.)* Before a child begins to talk, he uses a variety of vocalizations to express himself and to communicate with others. The 15- to 20-month-old child frequently emits long vocalizations that are qualitatively differentiated to communicate discomforts such as hunger, pain, or fright. Vocalizations of very young infants generally consist of vowel sounds. Most children master all the vowel sounds of American English by the age of 3 to $3\frac{1}{2}$ years. Consonants emerge in hierarchical order as mastered phonemes between ages 3 and 7. Some consonants are more difficult to produce than others and are mastered later in the development sequence. The first words spoken are usually nouns.

218. The answer is D. *(Hazzard, 3/e, pp 1016–1017.)* There are significant changes in cognitive and physiologic functioning that develop with age. Most studies of aging use cross-sectional methods, which usually show greater age-related declines than do longitudinal methods, which show the age-related declines to occur at an older age. The result has been to recognize that there is a great degree of individual variability to be found in cognitive and in physiologic functioning. Inter- and intraindividual variability have been found to increase with aging. Therefore, group or normative data do not reveal results as valid as those of longitudinal data, nor are group norms or cross-sectional data as valid a measure of an individual's variability. For example, various cognitive abilities show a decline in the group means in cross-sectional studies, whereas longitudinal studies show individuals to experience cognitive decline at different ages and at different rates. One's life-style and educational, intellectual, and other growth experiences have been found to play a major role in the retention or delayed decline of various cognitive functions. Tests of sustained attention show that the elderly perform extremely well into old age with less than one standard deviation of change between ages 20 and 80.

219. The answer is D. *(Hazzard, 3/e, pp 125–141, 154, 177–184.)* A major problem in attempting to provide health care for the elderly is understanding and counteracting some of the common stereotypes of aging. Although it is generally true that all five senses tend to decline in old age, it is not true that most old people feel miserable most of the time. In fact, recent studies show that the majority of the aged see themselves as being as happy as they were when they were younger. Boredom and lack of meaningful activity do become major factors with some aged, however. Another misconception is that a high percentage of the aged population live in long-stay institutions, such as nursing homes, mental hospitals, and homes for the aged. Actually, only about 5 percent of persons 65 and over, and about 10 percent of persons age 75 and over, are in long-stay institutions. Attempting to retain one's social, physical, and cognitive independence is a dominating factor and priority among the aged. Also, contrary to the stereotype that older drivers have a high automobile accident rate, older drivers have about the same accident rate per person as middle-aged drivers and a lower rate than drivers under age 30. By age 85, however, the crash rate is highest per mile driven. Longitudinal research has demonstrated that personality traits are highly stable after about age 30.

220. The answer is A. *(Hazzard, 3/e, pp 3–16.)* In spite of advances in medical science, there has been no extension of the limit of the life span, although a greater proportion of the population is reaching the apparent biologic limit of 85 plus or minus 10 years. It is estimated that life expectancy would increase only about 20 years if all heart disease and cancer were eliminated. In effect, prevention and intervention have improved cohort survival as specific causes of fatal diseases have been conquered. In general, the risk of death in the elderly increases exponentially with time. However, the biomedical model for diseases is not as applicable today since death increasingly occurs in the absence of disease. One series of studies has shown that some cells are apparently programmed for a fixed and limited number of reproductions, and then they die. This has provided some new concepts on aging and death. The $\dot{V}_{O2max}$ has been determined to be an integrated measure of the functional limits of the whole body. Furthermore, the relative impairment and functional age of a person can be evaluated by the use of a simple nomogram.

221. The answer is E. *(Schuster, 3/e, pp 281–293.)* Over the past 2 decades, many programs have attempted to improve the school performance of children from lower-class or disadvantaged homes. Most such studies have focused on developing competencies and motivational patterns that would provide the skills necessary to improve cognitive and academic performance. In general, they have demonstrated considerable success in improving subsequent cognitive and academic performance, including IQ. The degree of success is most often related to instituting the educational stimulation as early as possible; focusing directly on cognitive, language, and number skills; maintaining the effort over a prolonged period of time (years); and providing the stimulation on a daily basis rather than occasional exposure. These studies have also shown the importance of working with the powerful forces exerted on children by the values of the family and the community and the patterns of identification with social class and ethnic groups. A few isolated months or years of intervention cannot always offset the conditions and influences of the socioeconomically disadvantaged child. Programs that have been declared as unsuccessful in enhancing the intellectual functioning and academic success of such disadvantaged children have most often failed to provide one or more of the four listed components.

222. The answer is D. *(Lerner, Psychology, pp 446–453.)* Children born to adolescents are more likely to be of low birth weight than children born to older women. These children also have higher rates of infant mortality, mental retardation, and birth defects. All the tendencies apply across different races. Pregnant adolescents are also less likely to have had adequate prenatal care, the maternal death rate for adolescents is higher, and they are more apt to suffer from medical complications such as toxemia and anemia and from poor nutrition. They are also more apt to suffer from a higher degree of poverty and have a limited economic and educational future.

223. The answer is E. *(Hazzard, 3/e, pp 102–112.)* Although significant developmental changes continue to occur throughout adulthood, there is an increasing range of differences, or variability, between individuals of the same chronologic age. Hence, there are no predominant and universal developmental stages in adulthood as one finds in childhood and adolescence. Even if such predominant stages could be defined, the age at which people experience such stages or the sequence in which they occur is much more variable. In adulthood, changes occur in all areas of development (cognitive, physical, and social-personal). These changes may be a quantitative change in level, rate, or degree or a qualitative change in the nature or type. Thus, an aging adult's level of performance on an ability test may be reduced quantitatively, but qualitatively different forms of intelligence unique to adulthood, such as wisdom, may be acquired. Positive growth and change are expected and encouraged in childhood and adolescence, but in adulthood society does not provide such expectations and encouragement. The full potential for adult development has not begun to be realized.

224. The answer is B. *(Rosen, pp 205–214.)* In general, there is a gradual improvement of health behaviors with age. In children 8 to 15 there is a decline in health behaviors with decreasing regularity in eating and sleeping, and an increase in new risk behaviors such as smoking and drinking. In young adulthood, this pattern reverses itself with gradual improvements in health behavior, including eating habits. The health behavior that does not improve with age is physical exertion. This is unfortunate since lack of exercise shows the highest level of association with illness and mortality in the aged. In spite of the fact that older people report more symptoms, they also report themselves as being in more positive health status, especially people over the age of 60.

225. The answer is B. *(Rosen, pp 42–45).* Alcohol is clearly the most widely used drug by youth between the ages of 12 and 17, and the problem drinkers are more likely to use illicit drugs than are nondrinkers and typically exhibit other antisocial behaviors. These behaviors appear to make them more tolerant of deviance, especially since problem drinkers are less religious, less successful in school, and more concerned with independence than with academic pursuit. Traffic accidents, one-half related to alcohol use, are the most frequent cause of death and disability of youth.

226. The answer is E. *(Kandel, 3/e, pp 946–947).* In the 1940s, René Spitz compared the development of infants in a foundling home (much less contact with other human beings) with those in a prison's nursing home (where the mothers were allowed to spend time with their children). Both facilities provided good medical care and nutrition. After 4 months the foundling home infants actually scored better on several developmental indices (perhaps a genetic influence), but by 12 months the foundling home children had fallen far below the nursing home children. Further, many of the foundling home children had developed an anaclitic depression, were withdrawn with little curiosity or happiness, and were prone to infection. The nursing home children were similar to children raised in normal families after 2 or 3 years—walking well and talking actively. Of the 26 foundling home children, only 2 were able to walk or speak, and they could only say a few words. Spitz's findings have been confirmed by subsequent investigators, demonstrating that social interaction with other humans is essential in development, and that severe social and sensory deprivation in early childhood can have catastrophic consequences for later development.

227. The answer is B. *(Schuster, 3/e, p 262.)* In order to assess the normal development of a child, it is important to understand the complex process and sequence of developmental skills that are involved in acquiring speech. Starting in the first 6 months of life, babies invent new noises and appear to experiment with them. Cooing usually begins around 2 months of age and occurs especially when the babies appear to be happy. By 4 or 5 months, babbling occurs. This is the practice of expressing alternative vowel and consonant sounds such as "baba." Babbling is an important skill to acquire before a child can learn to repeat sounds heard from other humans. Between 6 and 9 months of age, babies begin to repeat sounds or sound combinations that they have heard and advance to the lalling stage (chains of vowel sounds). Within the next several months, the babies attempt to imitate any and all sounds they hear. They begin to select those sounds that help them communicate their wants or that amuse them. Between 24 and 36 months of age, infants will be able to use 200 to 300 words in phrases and two-word sentences. By the age of 48 months, a child should have a vocabulary of about 1500 words that can be used in short sentences with almost 100 percent intelligibility.

228. The answer is D. *(Kaplan, 7/e, p 682.)* A person's sense of maleness or femaleness is known as gender identity. It is both biologic and social. One's biologic sex of physique, including external genitalia and genetic influence, interrelates with a complex series of rewards, punishments, parental and cultural attitudes, and gender roles to influence gender identity. Gender role behavior is learned and is also derived in part from gender identity. A normal and healthy developmental outcome requires a reasonable congruence of gender identity and gender role behavior.

229. The answer is E. *(Schuster, p 296.)* Significant gender-role identification and behaviors are learned early in life. Gender-related differences in play behaviors are evident as early as 13 months of age. Males are generally more aggressive in their play and problem-solving activities than are females. These early behaviors are apparently so critical to one's core gender identity that children who experience gender reassignment after the age of 2 are high-risk candidates for psychological disorders. Recent research involving choices in child play indicates that children 3 to 4 years of age are able to make gender-appropriate choices according to Western stereotypes. Three- to five-year-old male children appear to be more concerned about gender-appropriate play activities than are females at that age. This continues into adolescence, as adolescent males also appear to be more conscious of gender roles than are females of that age.

230. The answer is D. *(Rosen, pp 96–98.)* Puberty is associated with important biologic and psychological changes, especially in females with proliferation of fat cells, and general shifts in body image in reference groups from family to peers and in perceived identity. Parents attempt to exert considerable pressure to restrict adolescents' food intake, more so for girls than boys. Parents are unlikely to blame their sons for a weight problem but regard their daughters' obesity in terms of problematic eating behavior and actively attempt to restrain their eating behaviors. Attempting to apply strict parental restrictions on eating tends to minimize options for learning self-control skills. Daughters are generally more apt to eat in response to both negative and positive moods. Exposure to more restraint may lead weight-conscious females to regard the presence of other people as a signal for not eating or for eating smaller portions. Adolescent girls are more concerned with their weight and more apt to take drastic measures to control their weight (e.g., starvation diets or vomiting).

231. The answer is E. *(Schuster, 3/e, pp 680–687.)* While background variables of economic status, race, culture, housing, education, parity, and age may be more important variables in determining subsequent behavior of infants, the phenomenon of parent-infant bonding has recently been shown to be important also. The bonding that occurs during the critically sensitive period from the first hours and weeks of life has been shown to enhance such factors as language development, cognitive development, length of breast feeding (which may be both a cause and an effect), and touching and fondling by parents. The lack of parent-infant bonding tends to increase the amount of crying done by the infant, failure to thrive, and subsequent child abuse or neglect. While cause and effect may be interacting here, there are extensive animal studies that demonstrate the importance of biologic bonding. These findings have had a humanizing effect on physicians and hospital policies.

232. The answer is E. *(Schuster, 3/e, pp 537–546.)* Children identify with their parents because they want to and, involuntarily, because of a perception of similarities. Insofar as most parents are seen by a child as having desirable attributes (e.g., power, freedom, ready access to pleasures, mastery over the environment), the child, wishing to become the same, identifies with his or her parents. If the parents should provide such poor models that the identification process is hampered, the child is then likely to identify with other significant adults in his or her environment. Parental authority is a powerful force; obedience is quite different and distant from identification.

233. The answer is E. *(Conger, 4/e, pp 143–156.)* Many of the cognitive and personality changes that characterize adolescence may be related to the emergence of formal operational thought during puberty. Formal reasoning enlists cognitive structures that enables adolescents to subject real occurrences to speculative yet systematic thinking about probable consequences. Such thinking, essential to hypothetico-deductive methods, underpins certain adolescent views relating to idealism, romanticism, and egocentrism. The ability to infer what others are thinking and feeling (social cognition) actually becomes much more advanced during adolescence, in spite of adult perceptions that adolescents seem to be much less concerned with the feelings and thoughts of others.

234. The answer is E. *(Kandel, 3/e, pp 960–972.)* Recent evidence has shown that there are morphological and functional differences in the nervous system of males and females. It is known that hormonal deficiencies during early development may result in two syndromes: Turner's syndrome, an anhormonal state in which gonadal tissue does not form (resulting in a phenotypic female, but one who fails to show pubertal changes), and androgen insensitivity syndrome, which is primarily associated with genetic males. (This latter syndrome was formerly called "testicular feminization," but persons afflicted with it do not have feminizing testes and do not secrete estrogen-type hormones; they possess abnormal genes and are indistinguishable from phenotypic females in external appearance and psychosexual orientation and libidinal interests.) It is thought that this genetic disorder prevents or blocks responsiveness to androgens throughout development. It is also known that fetal exposure to heterotypical steroid hormones (hormones of one sex given to or influenced by the hormones of another sex) can cause hermaphroditism in genetic females, but it has not been demonstrated in genetic males. If, during the fetal period, the female fetus is exposed to an unusual amount of male hormone, the female organ development is distorted, partially reversing the differentiation of the peripheral sex apparatus. The adult sexual behavior of hermaphroditic females is also altered. Thus, the effect is not only on the differentiation of external genitalia, but also on the differentiation of neural tissues that mediate later patterns of sexual behavior. The developing nervous system of both genders is considered to be bipotential. While the female anatomic and behavioral patterns can develop in either an anhormonal or maternal-dominated prenatal environment, the active influence of androgens is required for the development of a male pattern. Furthermore, there is a critical time period during which specific interactions between the developing brain and its environment (internal and external) will mold neuronal and behavioral capabilities. There is increasing evidence that the effects of the perinatal male hormones upon subsequent sexual behavior are more upon the developing central nervous system than upon the peripheral sexual apparatus.

235. The answer is D. *(Schuster, 3/e, pp 223–225.)* Cognitive skills in children develop in a fairly predictable pattern. Most cognitive behaviors can be expected to emerge chronologically. In comparing average age with expected behaviors of early childhood, one can expect the average 18-month-old child to begin many questions with "what," imitate almost everything in his or her environment, understand space only from his or her own activity of moving through it, begin to follow simple one-part directions, and begin to infer causes from observing effects. The average 2-year-old child can be expected to begin to learn about time sequences (e.g., "after lunch"), may arrange several words together in grammatically incorrect two- or three-word sentences, matches simple shapes and colors, attempts new solutions to old problems, and demonstrates a beginning cooperation in toilet training by anticipating a need to "go." By the age of 3, the child can be expected to ask many "why" questions, talks in sentences using four or more words, may talk about his fears, can give his first and last name, and may explore the environment outside the home if given the chance; in addition many retain urine through a night's sleep and wake up dry. By the age of 4 years, the child begins many questions with "where," may talk with an imaginary playmate, may threaten to "run away from home," can give opposites (up-down, hot-cold, and so on), and can associate familiar holidays with their seasons. Asking questions with "how," knowing the days of the week, identifying coins correctly, and following a three-step direction in proper order usually do not occur until the age of 5 years. At 5 years, the child may also begin asking the meaning of words, talks more "constantly," and may need to be reminded to eat or go to the bathroom because attention is so externally focused that he may fail to recognize subtle internal physiologic cues. Knowing the average age at which certain cognitive skills can be expected to develop can be of great assistance in helping the physician monitor the normal, or typical, growth or development of individual children.

236. The answer is A. *(Conger, 4/e, pp 70–89.)* Growth spurts occur for both boys and girls. A growth spurt for girls usually has its peak velocity at about 12 years of age, whereas the growth spurt for boys will have a peak velocity at 14 years of age. Although the adolescent growth spurt for girls typically begins at $10\frac{1}{2}$ and ends at age 14, it can start as early as age $9\frac{1}{2}$ and end as late as age 15. Similarly, menarche can come at any time between the ages of 10 and $16\frac{1}{2}$ and tends to be a late event of puberty. The adolescent growth spurt of boys can begin as early as age $10\frac{1}{2}$ or as late as 16 and can end anywhere from age $13\frac{1}{2}$ to $17\frac{1}{2}$. Growth of the testes can begin as early as age $9\frac{1}{2}$ and as late as $13\frac{1}{2}$ and end at any time between the ages of $13\frac{1}{2}$ and 17. In the United States, the rate of decreased age of menarche has been about 4 months per decade.

237. The answer is E. *(Schuster, 3/e, pp 376–392.)* Although a child's discovery of death is a private and individual experience, it is closely related to cognitive and affective developmental stages. Cognitively, a child must be able to conceptualize animate versus inanimate objects, comprehend cause-effect relationships, and deal with concrete factors before dealing with the abstract. Affectively, sufficient ego-strength, separateness, uniqueness, vulnerability, and coping skills must be developed. The infant must develop a concept of self before being able to comprehend "me — not me."

Between birth and 2 years of age, the infant is aware of separation through object loss and separation anxiety. This deprivation is an early form of experiencing separation as something synonymous with death. Children 3 and 4 years of age believe that all things think, feel, and experience things as they do. Thus they think that a toy feels pain when it is broken and that it must feel hurt when it is repaired. Also, they consider death as another form of life. At 4 and 5 years of age, they believe that death is a cessation of movement but that the dead person or animal continues to experience feelings. Cross-cultural studies have identified many primitive peoples who conceptualize death on this level, since many of them place food, drink, and other objects at the grave or in the tomb of the deceased. Our custom of placing flowers and other adornments on graves may, in part, be a remnant of this level of conceptualizing death. Children at this age are also apt to associate death with retaliation or punishment, which may lead them to fear, anger, and aggression toward others. Physicians must be aware of this possible interpretation of the 5- and 6-year-old child as a reaction to death, especially in the child's own family.

At 5 or 6 years of age children are apt to feel that death can be avoided and that they are not responsible for another person's death. They also begin to realize that their own significant others can die, and this can lead to notable uncertainties and insecurities. Children at 7 to 9 years of age begin to accept the inevitability of death for all living things, but believe that somehow it is external to oneself. By 10 or 12 years of age, death begins to be accepted as a biologic finality and understood in relation to natural laws, rather than being perceived as the result of aggression or trauma. Children at this age can see illness and accidents as causative agents and also that death originates within us and is not just external to us. No longer does the child feel that the dead person continues to live and feel in the grave. Adolescents spend much time in abstract thought about death and try to integrate the past, present, and future experiences into a philosophy of life. They still find it difficult to accept the concept of nonexistence, and this difficulty may extend into adulthood or even old age.

238–241. The answers are 238-D, 239-A, 240-C, 241-B. *(Schuster, 3/e, pp 194–195.)* The development of both gross and fine motor skills has been clearly observed and scientifically documented for various ages and stages of development. At the age of 18 months, a child can run, climb, throw a small ball, drink from a cup without much spilling, turn several pages of a book together, unzip a large zipper, scribble with a pencil, and build a tower of four or five blocks.

At 2 years of age, a child can try to jump, can turn doorknobs that can be reached, can drink from a small cup using only one hand, turn pages of a book one at a time, unbutton large buttons, and build a tower of six or seven blocks.

At 3 years of age, a child can peddle a tricycle, jump from a low step, begin to use blunt scissors, copy a circle, wash hands and brush teeth (but not adequately), and imitate a bridge made of three blocks.

At age 4, a child can hop forward on one foot, walk backward, cut around pictures with scissors, copy a square, button side buttons, and may bathe with assistance.

At 5 years of age, a child can jump rope, stand up without using hands, may be able to print own name, copy a triangle, dress without assistance, eat with a fork, and put toys away neatly.

242–244. The answers are 242-C, 243-A, 244-E. *(Schneiderman, pp 257–275, 547–548.)* A person's developmental level directly affects cognitive, social, emotional, and behavioral factors in illness. Chronologic age is of less value to the health professional in assessing and anticipating problems in treatment and prevention. Persons with mental or physical handicaps can be particularly difficult to assess and predict.

Preschool children generally see being sick as the result of some external agent (e.g., germs). They believe that getting well depends on strict adherence to rigid health rules. They are also more apt to view hospitalization as a punishment for bad behavior. This makes preparatory procedures especially important prior to and during hospitalization in order to deal with anxiety and stress. Because of close ties between the preschool child and parents, separation from parents can be an extreme source of stress for both the child and the family.

In adolescence, the complexities of illness and health and the more sophisticated interaction of internal and external factors become more prominent. The long-range consequences of an illness are not apparent, however, and the adolescent views himself or herself as indestructible or immortal. Peer group activities are of extreme importance. Adolescents will deny or neglect their medical care or health so as not to appear "different." Diabetes provides special difficulties. Peer pressures to drink or smoke can also undermine present or future health.

A major concern of the elderly is the possibility of developing a debilitating illness. The fear is that they might lose control of their mental and physical abilities and become dependent on or rejected by significant others. Other concerns are possible disfigurement or handicap, impending death, extended pain, chronic hospitalization, and invalid status.

Communication and Interaction

DIRECTIONS: Each question below contains five suggested responses. Select the **one best** response to each question.

245. Interpersonal relationship studies have concluded that the most critical element to assure compliance behavior in a physician-patient relationship is

(A) the exchange of accurate information and facts
(B) the congruence of expectations of physician and patient
(C) similarity of physician's and patient's age
(D) recognition and down-playing of social class differences between physician and patient
(E) allowing for the patient to be rewarded in some way for compliance

246. The type of information that is most effective in helping patients cope with anticipated surgery is information about

(A) procedures to expect
(B) complications that can occur
(C) sensory experiences to expect
(D) other patients' experiences
(E) medications before and after surgery

247. The first reaction of most patients when told they have cancer is

(A) the question "Why me?"
(B) an appeal to God or a higher power
(C) anger at oneself or doctor
(D) disbelief
(E) depression

248. Pretest counseling for the antibody test that diagnoses HIV infection is primarily directed at

(A) identifying the source of transmission to help others face the seriousness of the problem
(B) securing an extensive history for posttest follow-up and advice
(C) persuading both partners to seek help and treatment
(D) helping the patient to change his or her high-risk behavior
(E) recognizing and treating pre- and posttest stress

249. Your new patient is a 45-year-old, recently divorced woman. She has just told you that her 25-year-old son returned home 3 days ago with AIDS, and that she has experienced severe chest pains when she thinks about it. She starts to tell you about some other disturbing symptoms, begins to cry, and looks away. Of the following, which would be the most appropriate immediate response to facilitate the interview?

(A) Silence
(B) "I know how you feel"
(C) "Don't worry, it'll be OK"
(D) "Why are you so upset? You know you can tell me anything"
(E) "Are you thinking that you may have AIDS?"

250. The highest patient adherence (compliance) can be achieved by

(A) communication that is technical and authoritative
(B) the patient's belief that his or her health is influenced by internal control
(C) the patient's belief that his or her health is influenced by external control
(D) explanations of need for prophylactic medicine
(E) patients being treated for chronic disease

251. You are asked to see a middle-aged male patient who is complaining of frequent chest pains. As you enter the examining room, the patient is sobbing and blurts out, "My father died just like this 2 years ago." Your next step should be to

(A) reassure him that his pain is not related to his father's illness
(B) get more information on how his father's pain manifested itself
(C) order an emergency electrocardiogram
(D) introduce yourself and inquire about family history of heart disease
(E) ask a sufficient number of direct medical questions to establish that this is not an emergency

252. In preoperative patients, which type or types of information will be most effective in reducing stress?

(A) Sensory information
(B) Procedural information
(C) Coping information
(D) Sensory and procedural information
(E) Sensory and coping information

253. In judging facial expressions, the most difficult emotion to recognize and differentiate in most cultures is

(A) happiness
(B) disgust
(C) sadness
(D) surprise
(E) anger

254. The intervention style that is most effective in relieving the stress of surgery and enhancing the outcome is to provide the patient with

(A) problem-focused information
(B) emotion-focused information
(C) a match between personality factors and treatment style
(D) maximum family support
(E) as much preparatory medical information as can be understood

255. Which of the following interventions has been found to be most effective in reducing preoperative distress and facilitating recovery?

(A) Procedural information
(B) Reassurance
(C) Interpersonal support
(D) Hypnosis
(E) Relaxation training

256. Which of the following is considered the most powerful nonverbal communication?

(A) Touch
(B) Gesture and posture
(C) Dress and grooming
(D) Physical distance
(E) Facial expression

257. The length of the typical physician-patient interaction time is

(A) correlated with patient satisfaction
(B) positively correlated with patient compliance
(C) about 15 min for office-based specialists
(D) about 15 min for office-based internists
(E) about 15 min for office-based pediatricians

DIRECTIONS: Each numbered question or incomplete statement below is NEGATIVELY phrased. Select the **one best** lettered response.

258. In opening an initial interview with a patient, the LEAST important thing to do is

(A) ask the patient why he or she has come
(B) state what you already know concerning the problem
(C) refrain from duplicating questions already gathered in the chart
(D) ask open-ended questions
(E) project an image of authority

259. Mothers rate their satisfaction with their children's physicians as higher when the physicians are seen as demonstrating each of the following EXCEPT

(A) understanding
(B) provision of information the parents expect
(C) good communication skills
(D) efficiency and businesslike demeanor
(E) caring

260. In informing a patient or a patient's relative of the patient's serious illness, it is LEAST important to

(A) establish clearly that you would prefer to talk about it only after you have all the facts, tests, and other relevant information
(B) find out what the person thinks or knows about the illness
(C) find out what the person wants to know about the illness
(D) give honest answers in such a way as to leave the person with some realistic hope
(E) determine the person's understanding of what you have discussed

261. Statements about patients' or physicians' perceptions of symptoms that are generally true include all the following EXCEPT

(A) physicians tend to focus on symptoms that have serious implications for future health
(B) physicians usually focus on symptoms according to visibility or recognizability
(C) patients often focus on symptoms that interfere with usual activities or routines
(D) patients tend to focus on the degree of discomfort rather than the amount or degree of tissue damage
(E) patients tend to deny symptoms they fear may be related to a severe illness

262. Common attitudes and feelings of others about cancer patients include all the following EXCEPT

(A) fear they might catch the disease
(B) tendency to attribute disease to past behavior or undesirable traits of the patient
(C) fear that discussion about cancer will make the patient uncomfortable
(D) ambivalent feelings about patients with cancer
(E) feeling that they should tell the patient the "truth" about their prognosis

263. Patients who are ill are LEAST likely to use denial when

(A) they view their social roles and expectations to be threatened
(B) they have detected symptoms that they fear to be potentially serious and life-threatening
(C) their fears are not matched by their capacities to take meaningful action
(D) there is increased opportunity for secondary gain
(E) they view their personal desires to be threatened

DIRECTIONS: Each group of questions below consists of lettered headings followed by a set of numbered items. For each numbered item select the **one** lettered heading with which it is **most** closely associated. Each lettered heading may be used **once, more than once, or not at all**.

Questions 264–267

Match the body language behaviors below with the correct interpretation.

(A) Not willing to enter into a communicative interaction
(B) Angry, hostile, or upset
(C) "I'm interested in you. Notice me"
(D) Assertive and domineering
(E) Submissive and fearful

264. Lower the eyebrows

265. Visually notice someone but then quickly withdraw visual contact

266. Cross arms and press knees together

267. Reach up and touch one's own throat

Questions 268–269

Match each situation with the appropriate learning mechanism.

(A) Operant conditioning
(B) Modeling
(C) Stimulus control
(D) Biofeedback
(E) Positive reinforcement

268. A young physician watches and imitates the behavior of an experienced physician who is interviewing a patient

269. A patient is able to modify his or her own heart rate and blood pressure by monitoring the readings from the blood pressure cuff

Questions 270–272

Match the statements or descriptions below with the appropriate forms of nonverbal communication.

(A) Facial expressions
(B) Emblems or symbols
(C) Illustrators
(D) Self-manipulators
(E) Display rules

270. Movements involving one part of the body doing something to another part of the body

271. Body movements that transmit a highly specific message

272. Sex difference in recognition and use

Communication
and Interaction
Answers

245. The answer is B. *(Gatchel, 2/e, pp 185–190.)* Low rates of compliance appear to result from defective relationships between patients and health care providers. The most crucial element in the physician-patient relationship is the nature of role expectations that each has and the congruence and mutuality of such expectations. The exchange of information and facts, similarity of ages, social class differences, and patient rewards are relevant at times but are usually of less importance than the congruence of expectations between the physician and the patient.

246. The answer is C. *(Kaptein, pp 24–25.)* Significant behavioral interventions have been devised to help moderate a patient's anxiety and distress over anticipated surgery or other threatening medical procedures. In addition to the patient's concern about the disruption of his or her normal routine, travel to the hospital, time off from work, child care arrangements, and so on, there are very real worries about the surgical procedures themselves and their outcome. Information about the procedures to expect, complications that can occur, other patients' experiences, and medications that may be necessary are usually important and helpful to the patient, but studies have demonstrated that information about the sensory experiences that will be or can be associated with the procedure is the most helpful. This allows patients to evaluate the threats realistically so that they are not overwhelmed by unexplained and unfamiliar feelings and sensations that might be misinterpreted by the patient as dangerous sensory signals.

247. The answer is D. *(Sierles, pp 169–170.)* When patients are told that they have cancer, the first reaction of most is disbelief and denial. This is the initial reaction described by Kubler-Ross and also Weisman, who maintains that shock and disbelief are followed by a more existential conception of one's own vulnerability and such questions as "What does it mean?" and "What can be done?" In Kubler-Ross' scheme, other reactions follow: anger, bargaining, depression, and acceptance. According to Weisman, mitigation and accommodation, convalescence with the resumption of activities as much as possible, and recognition of decline and deterioration are the stages. As denial becomes increasingly more difficult to maintain, "preterminality" and "terminality" occur, where only palliation helps; this is accompanied by a "death watch" stage. Weisman's more existential analysis deals with the concept of an appropriate death with emphasis on care, control, composure, communication, continuity, and closure.

248. The answer is E. *(Sierles, pp 12–13.)* Counseling and psychotherapy regarding HIV infection is a communication skill that every physician should have to help manage the major problem of stress and reduce suffering. The skill is similar to that required for patients with cancer or other life-threatening and terminal diseases. In HIV pretest counseling, the physician should be able to explain the meaning of the test and assess the patient's physical, emotional, social, and mental strengths so that the patient and the physician will be able to anticipate the patient's emotional responses and reactions in the event the test is positive. In posttest counseling, the physician should review the meaning of the test, reduce immediate distress, encourage open responses, reinforce strategies of behavioral change (whether the results are seronegative or seropositive), and review medical and psychosocial potential. Subsequent concerns will include deciding whom to tell; establishing a support network; building on the coping skills, attitudes, and perceptions of the patient; and engaging in appropriate stress-reduction training.

249. The answer is A. *(Sierles, pp 182–184.)* There are a number of ways a physician can facilitate an interview, but in this case momentary silence would be most appropriate; i.e., you should continue to listen and perhaps offer a tissue, a nod, or a simple affirmation of understanding her import, such as "I see." This would do more to support her by letting her express her feelings and not interrupt her flow of thoughts with another question or statement. Studies show that doctors tend to interrupt a patient after about 18 seconds, and that crying is very upsetting to many doctors, who then feel compelled to say something—anything. Statements such as "I know how you feel" are usually inappropriate because most doctors do not know how a patient feels (unless they have had a son come home with AIDS). "Don't worry, it'll be OK" is a shallow response and does not support or help the patient, as the patient realizes that the doctor does not know that the patient will be fine. The question "Why are you so upset" is often interpreted as an accusation or inability to understand or express empathy. Saying "You know you can tell me anything" may be an attempt to reassure the patient, but it is inappropriate in a new patient who does not know that you can be told everything at this point in the relationship. The question "Are you thinking you may have AIDS?" is an inappropriate interruption and a very unlikely guess as to what may be upsetting the patient. It could be appropriate later in the interview, but only after exploring many other physical and psychological factors.

250. The answer is B. *(Kaptein, pp 21–23.)* Some studies have shown that about 50 percent of patients fail to follow advice or treatment prescribed. The lowest rates for adherence (compliance) are found in situations where prophylactic medication or advice is prescribed, especially for patients with chronic diseases. Significant levels of nonadherence occur where the symptoms are not seen or felt by the patient and there are no immediate adverse consequences experienced, e.g., in glaucoma, lung cancer, diabetes, or hypertension. The quality of the patient-physician communication is one of the most important factors; the highest adherence occurs when the communication is more open and shared with sufficient opportunities to discuss ideas and concerns. Adherence is low when the information presented is extensive, complicated, technical, and easily forgotten or misunderstood. Another important factor is patients' perceived control of their own health matters (locus of control). There is less adherence if patients feel that they have almost no control and that their health is primarily influenced by external factors, powerful others, or chance. Adherence is higher if patients believe that they have a high degree of internal control and can take responsibility for their own health.

251. The answer is D. *(Sierles, pp 181–184.)* In an initial interview with a patient it is important to give a high priority to establishing a good doctor-patient relationship in order to facilitate good communication. With this patient it is important to introduce yourself, as this can have a calming effect on an emotionally upset patient if it is done in a reassuring and confident tone of voice. Since this patient is upset and has already told you that his father died with similar symptoms only two years ago, it is probably best to calmly inquire about family history of heart disease. Usually, such a patient will begin to calm down, will address your question, and you will have begun to establish a good cooperative doctor-patient relationship with positive communication. Immediately attempting to reassure the patient that his pain is not related to his father's illness is apt to be aggravating, since he will surmise that you don't really know that. Inquiring about his father's pain is not immediately helpful in reaching your diagnosis, and ordering an emergency electrocardiogram is premature at this point. Asking a number of direct medical questions is also premature for an excited patient until after you have established a more stable communication.

252. The answer is E. *(Gatchel, 2/e, pp 167–170).* Sensory information alone (what one can expect to feel) has been found to be the most effective type of information. Coping information (e.g., teaching coping skills, ways to relieve pain and discomfort) is the next most effective because it provides the patient with some sense of control. Procedural information (what procedures will be done) makes the surgery more predictable, but does not address the sensations one should expect. The most effective reduction of stress is achieved by combining sensory and coping information so that the patient is able to predict when pain will occur, how it will feel, and how to cope with it. Studies confirm that it is important for the patient to be able to establish or retain some sense of control.

253. The answer is D. *(Vander Zanden, 4/e, pp 89–91.)* Basic emotions, as expressed by facial behavior, are relatively constant across cultures. Of the six basic emotions—happiness, sadness, anger, surprise, disgust, and fear—all the different facial expressions can be recognized and differentiated across cultures except surprise and fear, which appear to be very similar. Even though different cultures establish and teach their own "display rules" that regulate the expression of various emotions, it appears that the central nervous system of humans is genetically prewired for the expression of emotions through certain facial behaviors (fixed motor patterns). Thus, the face is a very important vehicle for the nonverbal expression of human experience and emotion.

254. The answer is C. *(Gatchel, 2/e, pp 174–177.)* Attempts to match a patient's personality style and treatment or health care style have been found to be most effective in minimizing the stressful situation of surgery and maximizing favorable medical outcomes. Patients are individuals, each with different personality dimensions and needs and with different coping styles. Extensive problem-focused information (informing about surgical procedures and sensations) will be helpful to certain patients but anxiety-producing to others. Likewise, some will respond favorably to emotion-focused information or technical medical information, but others will become anxious, confused, or upset. Family support is usually helpful, but again, it can become overwhelming. Listening to a patient and understanding a patient's personality and coping style will help the communication in this very complex process.

255. The answer is E. *(Gatchel, 2/e, pp 167–170.)* Behavioral intervention prior to surgery has been found to reduce both pre- and postoperative distress and to facilitate recovery. Various interventions have been compared, and it has been demonstrated that relaxation training among preoperative patients reduces distress and facilitates recovery more than hypnosis, interpersonal support, reassurance, or information about procedure. Each of these interventions, however, has been shown to be more effective than no intervention.

256. The answer is A. *(Vander Zanden, 4/e, pp 71–92.)* All channels of communication between persons other than the literal meaning of words spoken are designated as nonverbal communication. All the following can be considered as nonverbal communication: gesture and posture; touch; dress and grooming; physical distance; facial expression; skin color (e.g., pale, blushing); body hygiene; and even voice inflection, tone, and volume. Nonverbal communications communicate more emotions and feelings than other types of information, and they are important in placing verbal communication into a context. Physicians must be especially sensitive to nonverbal communication in order to secure the maximum communication, information, feelings, and context. It is also important to recognize that differences in cultural and ethnic backgrounds are often expressed in different nonverbal communication patterns. Touch is considered to be the most powerful of the many forms of nonverbal communication as it can communicate such messages as caring, support, and intensity of feelings. It is also regarded as having significant curing power in its own right. Furthermore, touching can communicate valuable information to the physician about the patient, such as tension, temperature, anxiety, and muscle tone.

257. The answer is D. *(Rosen, p 344).* Physicians frequently claim they are limited by lack of time to spend with patients, and patients cite this as one of the most important factors in their decision to change doctors. Yet research does not support this contention. The length of the physician-patient interaction is not correlated with patient satisfaction. Also, there is a negative correlation between the length of the interaction and patient compliance with treatment, with the shorter interactions resulting in higher compliance, and longer interactions yielding lower compliance. One study indicated that the average time spent with office-based internists was only 8 min, and that across specialties the average time was only 15 min. Another study indicated that the average office-based time spent by a pediatrician was 5 min. While much time can be wasted with ineffective communication, such brief encounters may not be sufficient to address important behavioral data, patient concerns, and family history, which may be at the root of the patient's health problem (e.g., smoking, environment, diet, or stress).

258. The answer is E. *(Gatchel, 2/e, pp 200–202.)* The opening statement in initiating an interview with a patient is important and sets the tone as well as direction of the interview. It is important to learn directly from the patient why he or she has come and to state what you know in a frank and honest manner, recognizing the information the patient has given and encouraging a forthright relationship. The temptation to play the role of an authority may actually inhibit the exchange of information and encourage a dependency role. In general, one must look for interactions that facilitate rather than restrict the interview. Therefore, open-ended rather than yes-or-no questions will usually the patient to speak more freely, provide more information, and put the patient more at ease.

259. The answer is D. *(Gatchel, 2/e, pp 188–189).* Variables in communication were found to be most important when mothers consulted physicians about their children. Also, mothers rated their satisfaction as higher when they were provided with information and discussion that met their expectations, including an expected diagnosis or a discussion of causes of the illness. Physicians perceived as understanding and caring provided greater satisfaction, while those perceived as efficient and businesslike provided less satisfaction.

260. The answer is A. *(Isselbacher, 13/e, pp 2–6.)* Asking a patient "What do you think?" and then correcting or qualifying the answer is an important part of informing a patient or helping the patient to understand the illness and the prospects for the future. It is important to find out what the patient or relative thinks or knows or wants to know about the illness and to give honest answers that will leave the patient or relative with a realistic hope. It is also important to determine the patient's or relative's understanding of what you have discussed and to leave the communication channel open for further questions. A frequent error is for physicians to avoid giving any information or discussing the illness, especially the diagnosis or prognosis, by stating that they prefer not to talk about it until they have all the facts, tests, and so on. Many times the physician is fearful that he or she will only raise the patient's fear or anxiety or appear not to know what the illness is, or perhaps look bad in the patient's eyes by discussing the illness before all the data are in. Yet, the patient and family most often have a whole series of rational and irrational ideas about the illness and its prognosis that should be explored by the physician. The patient must know that the physician will be supportive, regardless of what he or she will be going through.

261. The answer is B. *(Last, 13/e, p 978.)* People evaluate and make decisions with respect to their symptoms according to a wide variety of influences. In general, two types of variables define a person's estimate of the impact of these symptoms: perceived seriousness and extent of disruptiveness. Physicians ordinarily focus most on symptoms that have serious implications for the patient's future health status. Patients more often focus on symptoms that tend to interfere in some obvious way with usual activities and routines and on the degree of discomfort rather than the amount or degree of tissue damage.

262. The answer is E. *(Lindzey, 3/e, pp 823–825.)* Cancer patients generally receive ambivalent responses from others in their own social support networks. Feelings are likely to be negative toward cancer patients and to arouse fear and feelings of their own vulnerability and the possibility they might catch the disease. People are often strongly motivated to protect themselves by attributing the disease to the patient's undesirable characteristics or past behavior. They also fear that any discussion about cancer or death or their negative feelings will make the patient uncomfortable. Therefore, they avoid discussing their feelings and try to assume a "cheerful" role. Under these circumstances, the frequency and quality of the time spent with the patient are most apt to decrease and a certain amount of anxiety is likely to be evoked. Because most people avoid discussing cancer, they will shy away from discussing a hopeless prognosis and will fall back into cheerful but irrelevant chatter that represents a tragic waste of what could be meaningful and quality time for both the patient and the family.

263. The answer is D. *(Gatchel, 2/e, pp 180–185.)* What patients know, believe, and think about their illness affects the symptoms they think to be important, what they see as serious, and what they think they should do. Their social roles and personal desires often lead them to deny an illness. They often ignore symptoms for a long period before taking action. Fear about particular illnesses that may be of life-threatening character often causes them to deny the existence of the symptoms or their seriousness. Also, when their level of fear exceeds their capacity to cope, denial is a very likely result. The psychological process of secondary gain will also produce a postponement of action but is not usually associated with denial. Health educators need to help people bypass the usual hypothesis-testing of the cause of symptoms and help them take action by consulting a physician.

264–267. The answers are 264-D, 265-A, 266-B, 267-E. *(Vander Zanden, 4/e, pp 83–91.)* A man may straighten his hair or adjust his clothes if he wants to signal "I'm interested in you" or "notice me." Likewise, a woman may stroke her hair, adjust her clothes, check her make-up, or push her hair away from her face. These are called preening behaviors.

If we feel positive toward a person we are more apt to lean toward them, stand closer to them, and look them more directly in the eyes. By looking a stranger in the eyes once or twice, we signal that we are willing to enter into some sort of communicative interaction. If we notice someone, look at them, but then quickly withdraw visual contact, we signal that we are emitting a negative signal that we do not wish to establish a communicative interaction. This has been called *civil inattention.*

We also perceive the lowering of brows as an assertive and domineering signal and the raising of brows as receptive and submissive.

The closed body position—holding in the elbows, crossing arms, pressing knees together—is a frequent signal emitted by persons who are apt to be angry, hostile, upset, or nonreceptive. In an open body position the elbows are held away from the body, hands and arms are extended outward, legs are stretched out, and one ankle is crossed over the other knee.

Submission and fear are also communicated by body language. The submissive role tends to be represented by such actions as crouching slightly, assuming self-protective stances, reaching up and touching one's own throat, standing pigeon-toed, or not sitting until the dominant person sits.

Physicians must be able to decipher a patient's body language in order to get the full message. Nonverbal patterns signal inner attitudes and feelings, and many researchers conclude that nonverbal cues provide a more salient and valid message than verbal cues.

268–269. The answers are 268-B, 269-D. *(Sierles, pp 75–79.)* Modeling—observation and imitation—is a very effective method of learning the practice of medicine and most other skills. We observe the behavior of another person, note specific aspects or details of the behavior, and then try to imitate the behavior. In learning to interview, physically examine patients, or perform therapeutic procedures, we practice and integrate our knowledge, as well as our observations of others, in order to learn and improve our skills. Modeling can also be used to help overcome a child's fear of surgery or to treat phobias. It can be used to produce negative results, as in advertising in which the macho aspects of smoking or violence are glorified. Positive uses of modeling might include observing another person with high status who demonstrates how to say "no" to peer pressure or how to find a nonviolent way to resolve a conflict or respond to an insult.

In the past it was assumed that people could not voluntarily influence their autonomic visceral functions. We now know that visceral functions can be conditioned. Continuous monitoring of visceral or muscular functions, e.g., with the use of blood pressure readings, the electromyelogram (EMG), or the electroencephalogram (EEG), will allow some patients to voluntarily influence (control) a visceral function, such as blood pressure and heart rate. This is called *biofeedback* because by watching the electronic data on the screen (feedback of a physical function), the person can complete the feedback loop by "willing" the increase or decrease of the function, watching it change, and maintaining the change. Biofeedback can be enhanced by combining it with such techniques as muscle relaxation. Contraction (tension) headaches can be relieved by using EMG feedback to relax forehead and temporal muscles; anxiety states associated with stress can be relieved by using skin temperature or perspiration measures and relaxation techniques. Also, blood circulation can be increased in the fingers through biofeedback and relaxation to relieve the symptoms of Raynaud's phenomenon. While biofeedback can be used to lower blood pressure, it is not as effective over the long term as relaxation, which can be used clinically for some patients with borderline or mild hypertension and without the need for antihypertensive medication.

Operant conditioning (also called *instrumental conditioning*) is a learning mechanism for increasing the probability of a response by introducing a reward or reinforcement.

Stimulus control is a clinical approach used in behavioral medicine and is based on manipulation of environmental stimuli responsible for initiating problem behaviors. In obesity, it may be necessary to remove "snack goodies," which can act as a stimulus to eat.

Positive reinforcement is the awarding or conveying of a positive reinforcer (e.g., peer approval or a special treat) in order to promote or ensure the continuation of a desired behavior. Modeling can also be enhanced (reinforced) if the teacher or peer provides approving comments or evaluations.

270–272. The answers are 270-D, 271-B, 272-A. *(Lindzey, 3/e, pp 283–285. Vander Zanden, 4/e, pp 71–92.)* The ability to read and interpret nonverbal expressions is of critical importance to physicians, since such expressions reveal both intentional and unintentional feelings.

Illustrators are movements that amplify or emphasize words as they are being spoken. These can be movements of the hands to illustrate or emphasize the emotion (e.g., easy or flowing versus jerky or rapid) or they can be facial movements, called *speech illustrators*, which usually involve the brow, forehead, and eyelids to accent, emphasize, or supply emotion to words being spoken. The type of illustrator used is often related to a person's ethnic background or culture. Clinically, depressed patients have a low use of illustrators; as their depression lifts, their use of illustrators increases. Other observations include the following: there is a decrease in use of illustrators when a patient is attempting to hide his or her feelings; as illustrators decrease, the average voice pitch level increases; and, in general, people who show a high rate of illustrators are regarded by others to be outgoing, sociable, and expressive.

Self-manipulators are movements involving one part of the body doing something to another part of the body. Examples include such movements as scratching one's head, picking one's nose, wringing one's hands, and licking one's lips. They differ from emblems in that they usually occur with little awareness and are not deliberate attempts to convey a message to another person. Also, observing them can be useful to the physician in learning more about a patient, although the message is often diffuse rather than specific. Anxious patients have a high incidence of self-manipulators, and self-manipulators are often regarded as an index of discomfort of a person ill at ease or tense.

Facial expressions, as a form of nonverbal communication, appear to be universal in both occurrence and meaning, particularly in regard to the six basic emotions of happiness, sadness, surprise, fear, anger, and disgust. Cross-cultural studies have demonstrated that people display similar expressions when experiencing a given emotion, even though there are cultural and other learned variations with regard to such dimensions as stoicism or intensity of emotional response that are governed more by display rules and that can mask or conceal universality of facial expressions.

An emblem is a gesture or movement that communicates a specific message or meaning within a given culture. In the United States the following are examples of emblems: crossing the index finger and middle finger as a sign of hope that something will happen or, occasionally, to indicate one is lying; holding the hand upright with the palm outward and fingers together and moving the hand toward another person to indicate "stop"; clenching the fist at shoulder level with elbow bent and moving the hand back and forth toward another person as a sign of protest, anger, or determination to "get even" or aggression toward the other person; forming a circle by joining the end of the thumb and the index finger while holding the arm upright to indicate "OK," or agreement. A wink is considered to be a facial emblem; a head nod "yes" or "no" is a head emblem; a shrug of the shoulders is a body emblem, and so forth. Emblems do vary from culture to culture, but the emotion conveyed is generally clear. One study found less than a hundred emblems for Americans compared with a few hundred for Israelis and Iranians.

A growing body of research demonstrates that women are generally superior to men in both the reading and transmission of nonverbal facial communications. This does not appear to be innate but is related to certain child-rearing practices in which girls are encouraged to pay attention to nonverbal cues and boys are actively discouraged. When comparing four different types of nonverbal cues (facial expressions, body movements, changes in voice tone, and discrepancies between different nonverbal cues), women were clearly superior in the recognition and use of facial expressions, but showed decreasing superiority with regard to body cues and voice tone, with about equal ability to recognize and use discrepancies.

Group Processes

DIRECTIONS: Each question below contains five suggested responses. Select the **one best** response to each question.

273. According to studies of attitude change, communicators can increase their persuasiveness by

(A) discussing only one side of an issue when an audience is hostile
(B) presenting only one side of an issue when a competing persuader will get a chance to present the other side
(C) discussing one side of the argument when it is not important to achieve long-lasting attitude change
(D) de-emphasizing their own expertise
(E) allowing an audience of limited intelligence to draw its own conclusions

274. The view that leadership is a reciprocal process of social influence with leaders and followers being influenced by each other is known as

(A) situational leadership
(B) contingency model
(C) social facilitation
(D) collective behavior model
(E) transactional leadership

275. Which of the following statements is true regarding a person's performance of a task in an isolated environment versus in the presence of others?

(A) Performance of all tasks is improved in social situations
(B) Performance of all tasks is impaired in social situations
(C) Performance of all tasks is essentially the same in social and solitary situations
(D) Performance is facilitated on easy tasks by the presence of others but impaired by such presence on complex tasks
(E) Performance is facilitated on complex tasks by the presence of others but impaired by such presence on easy tasks

276. The most successful primary and secondary prevention strategy against drug abuse has been

(A) an appeal to fear
(B) education regarding the dangers of drugs
(C) affective underpinning
(D) long-term hospitalization
(E) social resistance skills

277. Persons without social supports are more apt to experience

(A) longer life
(B) less practice of denial
(C) fewer somatic illnesses
(D) more dependency
(E) fewer crises

278. The Hawthorne effect is best illustrated by which of the following situations?

(A) Of a group of factory workers who volunteer for a study of productivity and piecework payment, more than 80 percent quit the project because of the influence of nonvolunteer workers
(B) A group of factory workers who volunteer for such a study demonstrate an improvement in work rate greater than that associated with changed working conditions because they feel specially treated
(C) Work rate increases when workers are allowed frequent brief rest periods
(D) Productivity increases when workers have more opportunity to participate in the organization of their daily routine
(E) Although many workers initially are reluctant to have their routines changed and are suspicious of managerial motives, such changes are quickly accepted if their connection with improved working conditions is demonstrated

279. Recent evidence has indicated that a person in a group will be perceived by its members as a leader if that person's communication is

(A) high in quality, regardless of the quantity
(B) high in quality and low in quantity
(C) high in quality and high in quantity
(D) high in quantity, regardless of the quality
(E) low in quantity, regardless of the quality

280. In the study of group behavior, deindividuation has been found to produce

(A) weakened restraints against impulse behavior
(B) ability to monitor or regulate one's own behavior
(C) decreased sensitivity to immediate cues
(D) concern about evaluations by others
(E) ability to engage in rational planning

281. Successful leadership is most contingent on which of the following?

(A) The leadership style of a particular leader
(B) The interpersonal relationship between leader and followers
(C) The type of task situation in which a leader is involved
(D) The amount of power available to a leader
(E) The training of the leader

282. One might expect the socio-emotive leader in a group, as opposed to the task leader, to utilize primarily

(A) expert power
(B) coercive power
(C) informational power
(D) referent power
(E) political power

283. In a small group situation, departures from norms are most likely to be tolerated if

(A) the group enjoys strong leadership
(B) the norms have been stated frequently and clearly
(C) there is consensus and cohesion
(D) a dissenting member possesses resources or talents prized by the group
(E) the setting is private

DIRECTIONS: Each numbered questions or incomplete statement below is NEGATIVELY phrased. Select the **one best** lettered response.

284. Accurate statements regarding changes that can occur in individuals' attitudes include all the following EXCEPT

(A) individuals strongly attracted to a group are less likely than other members to change their attitudes in response to facts conflicting with group norms

(B) individuals are more likely to change a privately held attitude than a publicly disclosed one

(C) attitude change is more likely to occur if individuals participate in a group discussion than if they listen to lectures

(D) the influence of a group's attitudes on an individual is weakened only if more than one person openly disagree with the group

(E) a disliked person is more persuasive in writing than on videotape

285. Social support provides all the following EXCEPT

(A) a means for interpretation of situations

(B) a good substitute for engaging in health-promoting behaviors

(C) the ability for social comparison and validation

(D) models for behavior

(E) access to significant others

286. In an emergency, all the following variables will influence a bystander to help EXCEPT

(A) perception that the other person is intoxicated

(B) proximity to the other person

(C) knowledge of what to do

(D) few others in the immediate area

(E) male gender of bystander

287. Studies on attitude change show that people are LEAST strongly influenced by

(A) facts and information

(B) comparison of their own attitudes and beliefs with those of others

(C) their own personal and social needs

(D) the need to reduce unpleasant motivational states

(E) the attributes of the communicator who is recommending change

Group Processes
Answers

273. The answer is C. *(Vander Zanden, 4/e, pp 194–204.)* Hovland, Janis, Kelley, McGinnies, and McGuire drew a number of conclusions concerning effective communication. For instance, the most effective communicators are those perceived to have both high expertise and credibility. With very intelligent audiences, communicators are more effective if they let their audiences draw their own conclusions; with other audiences, they achieve more attitude change by stating their conclusions explicitly. One-sided arguments are most effective when audiences start out agreeing with the communicator or when there is little chance that an audience will be exposed to the other side of an issue. Although one-sided arguments may be immediately effective, the resulting attitude change is not always enduring. Nevertheless, the studies demonstrated that communicators can increase their persuasiveness by presenting one side of an argument when an audience is generally friendly, or when their position is the only one that will be presented, or when they want immediate, though temporary, opinion change.

274. The answer is E. *(Lindzey, 3/e, pp 501–504.)* The transactional view of leadership is of a reciprocal process of social influence. The leaders are both directing the followers and being influenced by them. The focus is on the perception of and the relationship between the leaders and followers. Other important considerations in the transactional model are whether followers perceive the leader's position as legitimate or illegitimate, whether leaders perceive their groups in a positive or negative light, and the nature of the task faced by the group. This transactional view relates directly to the doctor-patient relationship and aids in achieving optimal communication. It is much more complex and interactive than former views, such as the situational view it replaced. The situational theory regarded the task faced by the group and the general situation within which it must operate as the most important factors, rather than the personality traits of the leader or group members as even earlier theories had proposed. The contingency model of leadership analyzes effective leadership in terms of two major factors: the leader's personal traits or characteristics and certain features in the situation that play an important role in the leadership process. This model is consistent with the transactional view but attempts to restrict the more fluid components by identifying task-oriented authoritarian leaders and contrasting them with less directive, warm, and relaxed leaders. The situational factors are the leader's personal relationships with other group members, the clarity of the group task, and the power of the leader over the group members. Social facilitation refers to the effects on performance caused by the presence of others; that is, the presence of certain persons can both facilitate and impair the performance of the group on a particular task. Collective behavior refers to the actions of unrelated persons who happen to be at the same place at the same time and who are responding to the same stimuli. Examples would be commuters waiting for a bus or train, persons fleeing a burning building, or persons at the scene of an accident. Under these conditions, group behavior and leadership may be quite different from that of organized or intentional gatherings.

275. The answer is D. *(Lindzey, 3/e, pp 492–496.)* Social facilitation has the effect, in minimal social situations, of improving individual task performance on easy or familiar tasks and of deteriorating performance on more difficult tasks. In general, social facilitation produces an increase in activation levels. Increased arousal level usually results in improved performance on familiar tasks but tends to inhibit the acquisition of new skills or performance on tasks that are complex and unfamiliar.

276. The answer is E. *(Last, 13/e, pp 778–780.)* Over the past 25 years, a number of programs for prevention of drug abuse have been tried. Even though most of them have a high "face validity," the appeal to fear, drug education, attempts to understand our affective selves, and long-term hospitalization have proved to be relatively ineffective in preventing initial or repeated drug dependency and abuse. The teaching of social resistance skills has been more effective than any of the other strategies. The development of general social skills for managing social interactions and overcoming social pressures to use and abuse drugs has shown 35 to 75 percent effectiveness compared (on 2-year follow-up) with 15 to 25 percent for other methods.

277. The answer is D. *(Lindzey, 3/e, p 859.)* Social support serves to buffer and protect healthy and ill persons from the negative effects of crisis and change. It also helps them with the coping and adaptation process. They live longer, have fewer somatic illnesses, possess higher morale, and have a more positive mental health. The physiologic impact of social support appears to affect cardiovascular disease; that is, it appears to affect positively serum cholesterol, catecholamine responses, and severity of coronary artery lesions. Most recently, an association has been found between social support variables and cancer. The pathophysiologic mechanisms mediating this relationship are not yet identified. Social support encourages independence and self-confidence and less denial since coping and adaptation are more effective.

278. The answer is B. *(Rosenthal, 2/e, pp 112–113.)* In a piece of classic research at the Hawthorne plant of the General Electric Company, it was found that participation by employees in a special research project had a greater effect on work output than did any of the changes in pay scales, rest periods, and working conditions that the investigators initially wished to study. This phenomenon, in which research participation has greater influence on behavior than do the particular manipulations involved in the investigation, became known as the Hawthorne effect. It suggests that one of the most effective forms of social influence results from making individuals aware that they have been selected for special attention. Such influence is used in a wide variety of social investigations, including most forms of experimental research.

279. The answer is D. *(Lindzey, 3/e, pp 505–507).* The more actively individuals participate in a group, the more they will be perceived as group leaders. This is found to be true regardless of the quality of participation, apparently because quality and quantity indicate different things to group members. Although quality gives some indication of the ability of the contributor, quantity is seen as an index of motivation. Persons who are regarded as highly motivated toward the group are likely to be perceived as the leaders of the group by its members.

280. The answer is A. *(Lindzey, 3/e, pp 27, 57.)* Deindividuation is a psychological phenomenon that exists in groups where the presence of many other persons appears to weaken the restraints against impulsive or wild behavior, such as destructive vandalism, mob violence, or looting. Their sense of self-awareness is reduced, thus reducing their restraints against impulsive behavior or decreasing their ability to monitor their own behavior. Anonymity, whereby a person feels submerged in a large, undifferentiated group, appears to be the most influential factor leading to a state of reduced self-awareness and deindividuation, thereby allowing the individual to engage in impulsive behavior. Other factors contributing to deindividuation are feelings of close group unity (which act as an external stimulus), a high level of arousal (which can be physiologic or emotional), and a focus on external events and goals (which detracts from or overpowers internal control and rational behavior). Various studies have demonstrated that the psychological results of deindividuation are a weakened restraint against impulsive behavior, inability to monitor or regulate one's own behavior, a lessened concern for evaluations by others, and a lowered ability to engage in rational planning and other cognitive processes. Studies also show that instead of blocking out or decreasing their sensitivity to immediate cues, as might be expected, people actually experience an increase in sensitivity and reaction to these immediate cues and their current emotional state.

281. The answer is B. *(Lindzey, 3/e, pp 513–516.)* In his contingency theory of leadership, Fred Fiedler presents three situational factors that are important for predicting both leadership style and who will be an effective leader. Of these factors, he considers leader-group relationships the most important, that is, whether the leader is liked by the members of the group. Another situational factor is the type of task structure—whether the requirements of a situation are clear or ambiguous, for example. To complete the definition of a leadership situation, the power available to a leader must also be determined.

282. The answer is D. *(Vander Zanden, 4/e, pp 444–445.)* Exercising influence on the basis of one's status as an expert may further successful completion of the task confronting a group but runs the danger of increasing the social distance between leader and group members, a consequence that would be of more concern to a socioemotive leader than to a task leader. Coercive power may achieve compliance, but only at the expense of a leader's rejection by the group. Informational power, like expert power, also would be more consistent with the task leader's purposes than with the socioemotive leader's, again because of the distancing produced by these power sources. Political power can be utilized with considerable persuasion but is distracting and can compromise a group's cohesion and motivation. Referent power, by appealing to shared elements among group members, generally tends to promote closer relationships between leader and follower than do the other forms of power. Thus, referent power is the primary form of social power available to a socioemotive leader.

283. The answer is D. *(Vander Zanden, 4/e, pp 218–234.)* Group members may wish to ignore a norm if it is burdensome or a source of punishment. Norm rejection is more easily achieved in the absence of enforcement and more readily tolerated if the rejecting member possesses strengths and abilities needed by the group. A norm that has been frequently and clearly stated is more difficult to avoid because members cannot then claim ignorance or misinterpretation. The threat of censure or punishment is a strong deterrent to violation of group norms, especially if the group is very cohesive and if the setting is one of privacy.

284. The answer is D. *(Vander Zanden, 4/e, pp 194–204.)* Publicly held opinions are much more resistant to persuasive effects than are privately held opinions. In his action-oriented research, Kurt Lewin argued that group discussion and decision-making are much more conducive to attitude change than simply listening to the same information from speakers and lecturers. Solomon Asch's dramatic research on conformity demonstrated that a majority opinion could lead an individual to give erroneous responses on very simple perceptual tasks. However, Asch also showed that this majority power could be considerably weakened by the presence of even a single individual who openly disagreed with the majority. Other investigators studying group influence have shown that members who are most strongly attracted to a group are least likely to be swayed by communications that are inconsistent with group norms. A likable communicator is more persuasive in changing attitudes if the communication is on videotape or audiotape rather than written. On the other hand, a disliked communicator is more persuasive with a written message.

285. The answer is B. *(Lindzey, 3/e, pp 820–826.)* Studies on the effects of social support have demonstrated that social support provides the ability for social comparison, for interpretation of situations and feelings, and for modeling behaviors and is a mechanism for access to significant others. Social comparison or social validation provides an important source of information on how others experience the same phenomenon. The social support group helps patients interpret their situation, their feelings, and what is happening to them. Members of a support group in a similar situation can also serve to model behaviors so patients can learn more about the meaning and appropriateness of their own behaviors. Support groups also provide easy access to significant others so that the patient can maintain and enhance personal relationships. Patients without social support are more apt to increase their reliance on drugs or other substances and have less motivation to engage in health-promoting behaviors.

286. The answer is A. *(Lindzey, 3/e, pp 956–959.)* Many people avoid taking action in an emergency situation. The farther away the bystander is and the more people present, the less likely is a bystander to get involved. One is more apt to help the more one knows what to do, the fewer people present, if one is a male, if the victim does not appear to be responsible for his or her mishap (e.g., stroke victim vs. drunk), if the negative consequences to the bystander are minimal and the positive consequences reasonable, if the bystander's freedom is not limited by helping, if the bystander is somehow forced to get involved, if someone else is acting as a helping model, and if the victim is dependent or without resources or has helped the bystander in the past. Altruism is most easily learned through positive reinforcement and imitation.

287. The answer is A. *(Vander Zanden, 4/e, pp 194–203.)* Many studies have been done on the impact of group influences on attempts to change people's attitudes and behavior. These studies view people as social beings with considerable dependence on others to provide them with knowledge about the world and about themselves. Persuasive facts and information are not nearly as effective in changing attitudes as are attempts to satisfy various personal and social needs, the need to reduce unpleasant motivational states, and the process of comparing one's own attitudes and beliefs with those of others. Other group factors that influence attitude and behavior include the communicator's credibility, the patterns of communication, and other attributes of the communicator and the situation.

Family and Community

DIRECTIONS: Each question below contains five suggested responses. Select the **one best** response to each question.

288. Adolescent delinquency in boys can be predicted most accurately on the basis of

(A) IQ
(B) physique or body type
(C) family size
(D) socioeconomic status of parents
(E) relationship with parents

289. Most mental health care authorities agree that the recent trend toward community-based treatment of patients who have emotional disorders, as opposed to their incarceration in public mental institutions, can be ascribed principally to

(A) improved therapeutic results when treatment is available within a patient's community
(B) the development of preventive measures for various mental illnesses
(C) the use of new drugs that allow many emotionally disturbed patients to function outside an institution
(D) an increasing willingness by general hospitals to accept mentally disturbed patients
(E) the 1961 report of the Joint Commission on Mental Illness and Health, which strongly recommended community mental health programs

290. A Stanford University community health education study evaluated the effects of an educational campaign on reduction of cardiovascular risk factors. One community was exposed to mass media education, another received both mass media education and behavior modification training, and a third served as a control group. The most impressive results included which of the following?

(A) Cigarette smoking, egg consumption, and cholesterol levels declined equally in both test communities
(B) The control community made important achievements
(C) The mass media campaign plus the behavioral modification training achieved the most significant results
(D) It is better to focus on one public medium of communication at a time
(E) The mass media campaign had the most impact

291. The most efficacious way to actually reduce automobile accidents and deaths among teenagers is to

(A) provide driver education
(B) raise the legal age for drinking
(C) increase insurance costs (increase the penalty for reckless driving)
(D) raise the legal age for driving
(E) require use of seat belts

292. The two main functions of the family in America today are considered to be

(A) socialization of children and nurturance and security of adult personalities
(B) achievement of economic security and regulation of sexual behavior
(C) socialization of children and regulation of sexual behavior
(D) achievement of economic security and perpetuation of lines of inheritance
(E) perpetuation of lines of inheritance and stabilization of adult personalities

293. The most common parental characteristic found in cases of child abuse is

(A) low tolerance for frustration
(B) employment of harsh mental punishment
(C) rejection
(D) parents treating the child as they were treated by their parents
(E) persuasiveness

294. Ethnocentrism is the

(A) belief that ethnic groups should remain geographically segregated

(B) tendency to think that one's own group or way of life is preferable or superior

(C) belief that ethnic groups should not intermarry

(D) belief that values held by marriage partners should be in accord

(E) belief that multiple cultural practices should be incorporated into marriage and the family

295. The percentage of married women who were employed rose from 5.5 percent in 1900 to what percentage in 1987?

(A) 26 percent
(B) 36 percent
(C) 46 percent
(D) 56 percent
(E) 66 percent

296. An early study by Pauline Bart looked at the "empty nest" syndrome. Subsequent studies of this syndrome have shown that women who have launched their last child most often report

(A) a less meaningful existence
(B) more feelings of depression
(C) less positive self-concepts
(D) less stress
(E) fewer social activities

DIRECTIONS: Each numbered question or incomplete statement below is NEGATIVELY phrased. Select the **one best** lettered response.

297. Effective parental discipline of children requires all the following EXCEPT

(A) consistency—no significant change in expectations should occur through time

(B) follow-through—parents should pay attention to the child's response to discipline

(C) immediate feedback—the quicker the consequences of an action are experienced, the more learning takes place

(D) self-disclosure—children need to know that parents are human and make mistakes

(E) corporal punishment—when accompanied by love, this is the most effective discipline

298. All the following statements about the development of independence during adolescence are true EXCEPT that

(A) sex differences in the age at which independence is achieved tend to be greater in societies whose economy depends on the male's physical strength and motor skills (e.g., hunting and herding versus food-gathering cultures)

(B) compared with the majority of other cultures, independence training in contemporary America begins relatively early but also is relatively protracted

(C) in general, the shift of parental attitudes toward permissiveness that occurs during adolescence is greater in fathers than in mothers

(D) in general, authoritarian parental attitudes are viewed by adolescents as more appropriate in fathers than in mothers

(E) confidence and self-esteem are enhanced by parental attitudes that encourage autonomy yet express interest in an adolescent's behavior and opinions

299. All the following statements about child abuse are true EXCEPT that

(A) fathers abuse their children more often than do mothers
(B) child-abusing parents often were abused by their own parents
(C) prematurely born children are more often abused than are normal-term children
(D) parents are more likely to abuse one "scapegoat" child than to abuse all their children
(E) younger children are more often abused than are older children

300. Which of the following hypotheses can LEAST account for reported inconsistencies between the attitudes people express and their actual behavior?

(A) Attitudes often are measured very imprecisely
(B) Norms, expectations, and situational demands can alter people's readiness to behave in accordance with their attitudes, while leaving unchanged the basic underlying attitude
(C) Attitudes are more often based on education and knowledge
(D) Attitude questionnaires often measure orientation toward some general category, whereas behavioral assessments often involve only one facet of that category
(E) Attitudes and behavior are reciprocally influential

301. Women with high rates of heavy drinking include each of the following EXCEPT

(A) young women with small children
(B) women with alcoholic husbands
(C) employed women in stressful occupations
(D) women with a high rate of amenorrhea
(E) women in the presence of men

302. The loss of a mate is often followed by a loss of all the following EXCEPT

(A) social validation
(B) decision-making responsibility
(C) task performance
(D) social support
(E) social protection

303. Research results show that all the following statements are true EXCEPT that

(A) married persons have a significantly longer life expectancy than nonmarried persons, especially when compared with formerly married persons

(B) separated or divorced men have a much higher admission rate to state and county psychiatric hospitals than do married men

(C) widowed women have a higher admission rate to state and county psychiatric hospitals than do widowed men

(D) widowed women have a higher admission rate to state and county psychiatric hospitals than do separated or divorced women and never-married women

(E) death rates for heart disease and cancer of the respiratory tract are twice as high for divorced white men compared with married white men

304. Absence of the father in the home has all the following effects on children EXCEPT that

(A) it has a more detrimental influence on the child's personality in early development than when the absence occurs after 5 years of age

(B) for male children, absence of the father because of divorce, separation, or desertion is not as detrimental as absence because of death

(C) for female children, the earlier the absence of the father, the more mothers are apt to display overprotection

(D) in cases of absence of the father because of divorce, adolescent girls actively and aggressively seek the attention of men

(E) in cases of absence of the father because of death, the reaction of adolescent girls is active avoidance of male peers and a preference for other girls as companions

DIRECTIONS: The group of questions below consists of lettered headings followed by a set of numbered items. For each numbered item select the **one** lettered heading with which it is **most** closely associated. Each lettered headings may be used **once, more than once, or not at all.**

Questions 305–308

For each description relating to community health, choose the factor with which it is most closely associated in the United States.

    (A) Personal income
    (B) Economic and social class structure
    (C) Age
    (D) Religious beliefs
    (E) Health beliefs

305. The nature and distribution of health care services

306. The overall health status of an individual

307. The widest gap between need and provision of health care services

308. The perception of patterns of disease and their relative importance

Family and Community
Answers

288. The answer is E. *(Conger, 4/e, pp 529–531).* The nature of an adolescent boy's relationship with his parents is the single factor most predictive of juvenile delinquency. In the most extensive study of the subject, J. G. Bachman found that the better a boy reported he got along with his parents, the less likely he was to engage in delinquent behavior. Other studies have found that delinquency is related to overly severe and overly lax home disciplines as well as to an atmosphere of mutual hostility and rejection between parents and children. Despite the widely held belief that most delinquents come from broken homes, recent evidence indicates that the incidence of delinquency among boys of unhappy, though intact, homes is greater than that among boys of broken homes.

289. The answer is C. *(Kaplan, 7/e, pp 201–205.)* The old approach of treating mentally ill people in large, isolated institutions is becoming outmoded largely because of the effectiveness of new psychotropic drugs that enable many disturbed persons to function normally. The success of these drugs resulted in the recommendations in 1961 of the Joint Commission on Mental Illness and Health to increase the use of community facilities in treating mental illness. Congress passed the Community Mental Health Centers Act in 1963 to provide funds for the construction of community mental health centers. As a result, general hospitals became more active in mental health therapy and community mental health centers developed to support mental patients in a functional atmosphere, in addition to taking steps at a local level to prevent mental illness. Cuts in the federal budget over the past 10 years have significantly restricted the programs and reduced the number of community health centers. As a result many of the patients who have regressed while in the community are not receiving the much needed drugs, social support, vocational counseling and training, a paying job, or psychiatric treatment. Thus, the potential benefits from new medications have been lost because of a failed public policy of deinstitutionalization.

290. The answer is C. *(Gatchel, 2/e, pp 306–307.)* The Stanford University community health education study evaluated the relative effects of an intensive multifactor health education campaign on the reduction of cardiovascular risk factors. The study developed a multimedia campaign to encourage people to lose weight, increase exercise, stop smoking, and change their diet. One town was exposed to a large-scale mass media campaign, another received the mass media campaign coupled with behavioral modification training for high-risk individuals, and a third served as a control community. Both test communities decreased cigarette smoking, egg consumption, and cholesterol levels. The community with the mass media campaign plus behavioral modification training achieved the most impressive results. The findings of the study clearly indicate that health beliefs and attitudes can be modified in natural settings as well as in research laboratories. Two problems were emphasized: the powerful countervailing pressures in society that promote smoking and eating of nonnutritional foods and the resistance to change created by the sedentary state of our highly automated society.

291. The answer is D. *(Rosen, p 16.)* While behavior change is most often the most effective means of promoting health, technological or regulatory measures can be more successful in certain instances. If the goal is to reduce automobile accidents and deaths among teenagers, raising the legal age for driving is more effective than driver's education or encouraging the use of seat belts. Raising the legal age for drinking or adding punitive insurance costs will have some reducing effect, but not as much as raising the legal age for driving. An aggregate strategy of mixing education, technology (safety devices), and regulation is the most effective.

292. The answer is A. *(Conger, 4/e, pp 160–189.)* The American family has progressively lost a number of its previous functions, such as educating its offspring and serving as a center of recreational activity. Two major functions are left to the family: socialization of offspring and stabilization of adult personalities. The influence of parents during their children's early years suggests that socialization is still one of the family's primary functions, despite the fact that other agencies (e.g., schools) have attempted to take over some aspects of this task. The second function, that of stabilization of adult personalities, is accomplished when men and women succeed in adjusting themselves to roles of parental responsibility and sharing nurture and security. The changes occurring in marriage, women's roles and child care and the factors of poverty, single-parent families, divorce, and remarriage are having a major impact on the socialization function, and particularly on the function of nurturance and security of adult personalities.

293. The answer is A. *(Schuster, 3/e, pp 246–247.)* Studies on child abuse have found that abusive parents have a common characteristic—a low tolerance for frustration. Also, abusive parents often use harsh physical punishment in controlling their children, which is usually counter-productive. Another repeatedly observed finding is that abusive parents tend to have been abused by their own parents. This creates a generation effect whereby the harsh discipline practices of one generation may serve as a model for the next generation. Thus physicians attempting to work on cases of child abuse should focus on breaking the cycle of parental behaviors for one generation. Many child-abusive parents may be rejecting and cold toward their children, but they are more apt to be overcontrolling than permissive.

294. The answer is B. *(Vander Zanden, 4/e, pp 409–410.)* Ethnocentrism is the tendency to consider one's group or way of life (usually national or ethnic) superior to other groups and to use one's own group as the frame of reference against which other groups are judged. Americans are sometimes considered ethnocentric because of the relative isolation of American families from persons of different cultures and their ways of life. This can often cause us to have a very narrow view of marriage and family life.

295. The answer is D. *(Last, 13/e, pp 571–572.)* In 1900, 20 percent of all adult women were in the labor force. Married women and women with children in the labor force significantly increased so that by 1972 there were 40 percent and by 1987 there were 56 percent in the work force. Fifty-six percent of married women with children are employed and married women with children under the age of 2 represent the fastest growing group in the work force. In 1950, 1.5 million families were headed by women, compared with 11 million in 1988, and 88 percent of these women are in the work force. The poverty rate of these families maintained by women is three times the rate for all families. The gender wage gap continues to exist and most women are still trapped in traditional women's jobs, which fosters job insecurity and job-related stress and health problems. These conditions are gradually changing for the better.

296. The answer is D. *(Kaplan, 7/e, pp 60–62.)* An earlier study by Pauline Bart argued that the role of full-time mother leaves women in a difficult and depressed state when their children reach adulthood and leave home. This was designated as the "empty nest" syndrome. Subsequent studies have shown that this conventional wisdom is misleading; that women report less stress; that many newlyweds visit or telephone their parents, use their cars, and so on; that with delayed marriage, getting children to leave home is becoming a bigger problem; that middle-aged women who had not launched their children reported much less positive self-concepts than those who had, especially in interpersonal relationships; and that, in general, women look forward to the freedom and opportunity acquired by having their children launched. The increase in divorce at this age is more often related to the departure's unmasking of an empty marriage than to the empty nest syndrome.

297. The answer is E. *(Schuster, 3/e, pp 343–346.)* The most effective parental discipline of children uses several basic principles that apply in all situations to all children. If properly used, these principles help children by guiding them toward the goal of becoming self-actualized, self-directed, socialized adolescents and adults. Parental expectations must be consistently maintained through time. The principle of follow-through entails parental attention to the child's response to discipline. If a certain form of disciplinary punishment is stated, then it must be carried through. Discipline should be paced with the maturation level of the child. The quicker the consequences of an action are experienced, the more learning takes place. This is the principle of immediate feedback. Delayed consequences are usually ineffective in changing behavior. Adults must be truthful with children at all times. Effective child-rearing practices involve mutual trust. Children need to feel that their parents are human and fallible just as they are. They need to know that parents often can and do make mistakes. The most important principle of discipline is genuine love. Adults and parents who really love their children rarely fail in raising autonomous, socialized, self-actualizing children. Genuine love is not an accident; it must be learned and pursued. Harsh physical punishment becomes counter-productive in that it relies too heavily on superior adult strength and develops fear rather than self-discipline.

298. The answer is C. *(Conger, 4/e, pp 195–212.)* Most societies stress independence more in male than in female adolescents; however, the sex difference is greatest in hunting and herding cultures. Independence training in American culture begins early but is prolonged, leading to the phenomenon that Erik Erikson has termed the "psychosocial moratorium." In contemporary America, parents usually shift toward more permissive attitudes as their child matures; however, this shift is more pronounced in mothers than in fathers.

299. The answer is A. *(Conger, 4/e, pp 194–202.)* Certain children are singled out for abuse by their parents; these children frequently were born prematurely and were slower to develop than were their siblings. Child abuse is committed most often on children below the age of 3. A principal finding in studies of the personality of parents who abuse their children is that such parents usually were abused by their own parents. Mothers abuse their children more often than do fathers, probably because mothers have more contact with their children. Most children who are abused come from poor homes and their families tend to be socially isolated. About 1 million children are maltreated each year; this maltreatment accounts for 2000 to 4000 deaths each year.

300. The answer is C. *(Vander Zanden, 4/e, pp 174–182.)* For many reasons, attitudes are never measured precisely. For example, test items may be ambiguous, or respondents may attempt to describe themselves in more favorable, rather than more accurate, terms. Behavior may be consistent with attitudes if situational norms and expectations favor consistency, but not if they do not. Researchers often use questionnaires that tap attitudes toward some general category, but measure behavior toward only one aspect of that category. Thus, a researcher might devise a scale to measure attitudes toward blacks, then ask respondents to pose for a picture with a specific black person. In a recent discussion of the attitude-behavior controversy, H. A. Alker has suggested that consistency may itself be an individual variable—that is, some people may show more consistency between attitude and behavior than others. In general, attitudes influence and are influenced by three components: the cognitive, the affective, and the behavioral.

301. The answer is E. *(Rosen, p 39.)* Studies of the drinking habits of women have found that the highest rates of heavy drinking are among young women with small children, women with alcoholic husbands, and employed women, especially women in stressful occupations. On the average, women tend to drink less than men, but in the presence of men they tend to drink even less. Effects of high ethanol intake particular to women include amenorrhea, decreased size of ovaries, absence of corpora lutea with associated infertility, and spontaneous abortion.

302. The answer is B. *(Lindzey, 3/e, pp 823–825.)* There is an increase in mortality following the loss of a mate and the subsequent bereavement. The loss of a partner leads to a deficit in the areas of social validation, social support, task performance, and social protection. The loss of social validation means loss of support for one's confidence in one's own judgments, assessments, and appropriateness of ideas and behavior. The survivor also recognizes the loss of routine and special tasks that were provided by the deceased. The loss of social support and unconditional positive regard seriously reduces a major source of self-esteem and self-regard. Not only is there a great deal of disruption, but it often fosters a sense of helplessness. Decision-making responsibility is increased, even though a sense of helplessness may occur. There are dramatic increases in health risks, such as those of suicide, accidents, alcohol and drug dependency, and tuberculosis.

303. The answer is C. *(Last, 13/e, pp 687–695.)* There are significant relationships between marital status and health status. The married have a significantly longer life expectancy than the nonmarried, especially when compared with the formerly married (widowed, divorced, or separated). Married persons have less chronic illness, especially mental illness, than the formerly married and make fewer requests for health care service. Children raised in single-parent families have more illness and make more demands on the health care service system than children in families where both parents are present. Death rates comparing divorced and married white men show that divorced white men have twice as many deaths from heart disease and cancer of the respiratory tract as married white men. Separated or divorced men have a higher admission rate to state and county psychiatric hospitals. Widowed men have a higher admission rate to state and county psychiatric hospitals than do widowed women, but widowed women have a higher admission rate than separated or divorced women and never-married women.

304. The answer is B. *(Lerner, Psychology, pp 596–598.)* Research on factors that influence children's personality development has often been directed at studying the effects of the absence or withdrawal of specific factors. Thus, to understand the effects of the absence of the father from the home, situations of separation, desertion, divorce, or death have been studied. Results have shown that the effect on the child's personality depended on the sex of the child and the timing of and reason for the father's absence. A father's absence during a child's early development has a more detrimental effect than when the absence occurs after the child is 5 years old. For males, the absence of the father caused by death is not as detrimental as absence caused by divorce, separation, or desertion. For females, absence of the father caused by death seemed to interfere more with overall adjustment than for males. Absence of the father alters the interaction of adolescent girls with other males, producing one of two extreme reactions. In cases of absence caused by divorce, girls actively and aggressively seek social and physical attention of men. In cases of absence caused by death, however, girls are more apt to react with avoidance of male peers and a preference for other girls as companions. Other studies have shown that the absence of fathers from either divorce or death caused girls to express more insecurity about their ability to relate to males; divorce more often led to overinvolvement, and death typically led to avoidance. Also, the earlier the absence of the father had occurred, the more mothers were likely to have displayed overprotection. Other studies of boys with absent fathers showed a tendency for conflict and uncertainty as to appropriate masculine orientations—sometimes resulting in a "supermacho" role as overcompensation and in other instances a more feminine orientation.

305–308. The answers are 305-B, 306-A, 307-C, 308-E. *(Williams, SJ, 3/e, pp 51–71.)* Several major characteristics of a community are directly related to health status and to health care systems or other approaches devised to meet perceived health needs. The nature and distribution of the present system of medical care in the United States are products of a political process determined in turn by economic and social class structure. These determinants of the health care system place power in a community's dominant individuals to decide how and to whom health services are distributed.

Personal income has a direct relationship to health. Such critical measures of community health as maternal mortality, prenatal and infant mortality, life span, disability, and hypertension are worse in all age categories among people who are poor. Unlike the affluent, the poor cannot buy good health services. When the data are adjusted for health status, the lower socioeconomic groups still have fewer visits to physicians than do higher socioeconomic groups. Primary care programs reach less than one-third of the medically underserved.

The elderly at every income level in every social class demonstrate a proportionally higher need for health services than do other population groups. Increasing expenditures for Medicare relate to increasing costs. The elderly and the poor continue to suffer disproportionate neglect on the basis of income, needs, and services available.

People's perceptions of their own health status can be influenced by sociocultural factors, including their particular community's technologic prowess. Indeed, all these factors shape a person's attitude toward health, an attitude that, in turn, eventually governs that person's response to his or her own health needs and use of the health services available. Level of education and income is related to the use of preventive services and preventive behavior.

Sociocultural Patterns of Behavior

DIRECTIONS: Each question below contains five suggested responses. Select the **one best** response to each question.

309. The F-scale developed by Theodore Adorno and coworkers was intended to be a measure of

(A) fear
(B) fixation
(C) frustration
(D) fascism
(E) none of the above

310. The risk for hypertension is greatest among

(A) whites of lower socioeconomic status
(B) blacks of lower socioeconomic status
(C) whites of higher socioeconomic status
(D) blacks of higher socioeconomic status
(E) upwardly mobile middle-class whites

311. Biologic responses are most adversely influenced over time by

(A) regressiveness
(B) interpersonal conflict
(C) confusion
(D) uncontrollability
(E) fearfulness

312. An important therapeutic aspect of *curanderismo* often lacking in Western scientific medicine is the

(A) ability to "cure" psychosomatic illnesses
(B) cultural congruence between healer and patient
(C) extensive use of symbolism
(D) laying on of hands
(E) use of herbal preparations

313. A *social norm* is best defined as

(A) a rule
(B) average behavior
(C) an individual's expectations of another
(D) shared expectations about behavior
(E) recommended behavior

314. The most effective method of reducing racial prejudices in an individual is through

(A) interracial contact
(B) introducing black studies into elementary school curricula
(C) psychotherapy for black-white confrontations
(D) improving the black image in the mass media
(E) campaigns to counteract stereotypes

315. A person becomes more vulnerable to conditions of psychological and physical distress if he or she is

(A) aware of results of diagnostic tests
(B) receiving medical information
(C) denying the illness
(D) introspective
(E) receiving counseling

316. Studies of pain response among different American ethnic groups disclosed that, for disorders of equivalent objective severity, the degree of open and vocal response to pain was greatest in which of the following groups?

(A) "Old American" and Jewish
(B) Italian and Jewish
(C) Irish and "Old American"
(D) Jewish and Irish
(E) Italian and "Old American"

317. Ethnic differences in response to pain are attributable primarily to

(A) differences in pain threshold
(B) differences in subjective experience of pain
(C) intellectual ability to grasp the significance of a disease
(D) cultural traditions of stoicism or emotionalism
(E) experimental bias

318. White Americans compared with African-Americans have a higher prevalence of

(A) hypertension
(B) insulin-dependent diabetes mellitus
(C) obesity
(D) tuberculosis
(E) coronary and cerebral arterial disease

319. The basic symbol of Chinese-American medicine is the

(A) mandarin hat and coat
(B) dragon
(C) dog
(D) snake
(E) yin-yang

320. The health belief model predicts

(A) morbidity of an illness
(B) mortality of an illness
(C) compliance with treatment
(D) risk of a patient
(E) whether a person will seek health care

321. Sickness is best defined as the

(A) patient's experience of not being well
(B) clinical diagnosis of disease
(C) laboratory diagnosis of disease
(D) medical labeling of a disease
(E) physician's perception of a disease

322. Higher socioeconomic status (SES) is positively correlated with an increased incidence of

(A) breast cancer
(B) coronary artery disease
(C) stroke
(D) lung cancer
(E) hypertension

323. Developmental research on gender-related differences has shown that females

(A) are more emotional
(B) have greater verbal ability
(C) have better visual-spatial skills
(D) excel in mathematical skills
(E) have less fine motor coordination

324. Among spiritual healers, the most common theory of disease is that

(A) disease is a spiritual malaise resulting from sinful acts
(B) disease results from psychological stress
(C) disease is caused by parapsychological phenomena
(D) disease is caused by germ-mechanical factors
(E) disease is caused by invasion of the body by evil spirits

325. True statements about reporting of symptoms and seeking help for them include which of the following?

(A) Women are more likely to report symptoms
(B) Men are more accurate in their reporting of symptoms
(C) Women are less likely to seek medical help
(D) Lower social status is associated with lower reporting of symptoms
(E) None of the above

326. Which of the following statements regarding pregnant adolescents is true?

(A) They show a positive relationship between weight gain of pregnancy and infant birth weight
(B) They retain nitrogen more efficiently than do pregnant adult women
(C) They have an incidence of growth-retarded children similar to that of pregnant adult women
(D) The birth weight of their babies is somewhat higher due to an excess carbohydrate diet
(E) Malnutrition in pregnant adolescents is rarely seen in the United States

327. Which of the following statements about infant mortality is true?

(A) Black infant mortality in the U.S. is about twice as high as white infant mortality
(B) Finland has one of the highest infant mortalities of all European countries
(C) Infant mortality in the U.S. is lower than in Canada
(D) Infant mortality in the U.S. is lower than in Spain
(E) Infant mortality in Hong Kong is higher than in the United States

328. In the 1930s, the smoking rate was 50 percent for men and 20 percent for women. In the past 60 years, cigarette smoking has followed different patterns for men and women. During this time the smoking rate for

(A) women has tripled over the entire 60 years
(B) women has now increased to the 1960 level for men
(C) women has increased at a steady pace over the entire 60 years
(D) men has been reduced to the 1930s level
(E) men decreased significantly between 1960 and 1990

329. The most effective strategy for reducing vehicular accidents during the 1980s was

(A) legislation
(B) education
(C) driver training
(D) safety engineering
(E) new technology

330. Studies on the sexual behavior of adolescent females show that

(A) the youngest are most likely to use contraceptives
(B) an adolescent who has had an abortion is more likely to be pregnant again within 2 years than one who has given birth
(C) parental involvement in a teenager's abortion reduces the probability of subsequent unwanted pregnancies
(D) each year about 40 percent of the 1 million pregnant adolescents obtain abortions
(E) median age for initiation of sexual activity is 14

331. True statements about poverty among older groups include

(A) poverty acts as a survival stimulus and helps to persuade the elderly to adopt a healthier lifestyle
(B) Social Security policy has increased poverty among older adults in the past 2 decades
(C) in 1984 more than 40 percent of older unmarried women were in poverty
(D) women are two and a half times more likely than men to be poor or near poor
(E) the life expectancy differential between lower and middle classes has decreased with Medicare

332. True statements regarding health beliefs include which of the following?

(A) The majority of people with hypertension are able to monitor their own blood pressure with signs and symptoms
(B) Patients assign more validity to their physician's instructions than to their self-assessment of their health
(C) Patients who believe they can control their health outcome are more apt to change their health-related behavior
(D) Younger patients are more apt to believe that controlling their emotions and staying mentally active are important preventive actions
(E) Older patients place more value on vigorous exercise to promote health and prevent illness

333. When the importance of social ties for health in the elderly is compared with that in younger populations, the elderly

(A) are more apt to experience significant life changes that separate them from social connections
(B) benefit increasingly from marriage as a factor that decreases mortality
(C) are more likely to maintain multiple sources of social contacts
(D) have less of a dependence on the support of friends and relatives
(E) are more stressed when not married

334. The factor most highly associated with the etiology of violence is

(A) family instability
(B) lack of education
(C) poverty
(D) crowded living conditions
(E) race

335. A 19-year-old Euro-American male in Miami has been shot by another 19-year-old male on the street in his neighborhood. The odds are that the shooter was

(A) Euro-American
(B) Asian-American
(C) Cuban-American
(D) African-American
(E) Mexican-American

336. Which of the following statements regarding suicide in the U.S. is accurate?

(A) It tends to decrease with age
(B) Rates for African-Americans are less than those for Euro-Americans
(C) Rates for females are two to three times as great as those for males
(D) It is attempted twice as often as it is completed
(E) Rates for poor persons are higher than for the economically privileged

DIRECTIONS: Each numbered question or incomplete statement below is NEGATIVELY phrased. Select the **one best** lettered response.

337. Behavioral signs and symptoms of alcoholism include all the following EXCEPT

(A) conservative religious practice
(B) problems on the job
(C) patterns of accidents
(D) marital difficulties
(E) driving-related difficulties

338. Dieting induced by social and cultural pressures results in all the following EXCEPT

(A) a raised basal metabolic rate
(B) hormonal changes that promote fat storage afterwards
(C) net long-term weight gain
(D) plateaus in the process of weight loss
(E) increasingly compulsive strategies in the pursuit of an ideal weight

339. All the following are characteristics of heavy alcohol drinkers in college EXCEPT

(A) they tend to come from large metropolitan rather than rural areas
(B) they are more likely to major in the social than the natural sciences
(C) they tend not to be deeply religious
(D) they use nonalcoholic drugs less frequently than nondrinkers
(E) their parents are more likely to use alcohol

340. In comparing the effects of consumption of alcohol on Caucasians and Asians, Caucasians exhibit all the following EXCEPT

(A) a higher rate of alcoholism
(B) lower levels of acetylaldehyde
(C) more reactivity of heart rate and blood pressure
(D) less subjective discomfort
(E) less facial flushing

341. Each of the following statements about minorities and the use of alcohol and the incidence of alcohol problems is true EXCEPT

(A) Asian Americans tend to drink less than non-Asian Americans
(B) rates of alcoholism among Hispanic Americans tend to be higher than the national average
(C) when American Indians enter an urban environment, the rate of alcoholism becomes much worse
(D) alcoholism among blacks appears to be increasing
(E) the incidence of alcoholism among homosexuals appears to be greater among females

342. Considering the characteristics of the population over age 65, all the following statements are true EXCEPT

(A) the older population has been getting larger
(B) the older population is expected to level off in numbers by the year 2000
(C) about 5 percent are residents of nursing homes
(D) the female population has increasingly outnumbered the male population
(E) of the 85-and-older segment, the number of men per 100 women is expected to decrease from about 45 to about 39 by the year 2000.

343. The basic technology of Native-American medicine uses all the following EXCEPT

(A) drugs
(B) surgery
(C) religious or spiritual practices
(D) blood-letting
(E) mineral springs bathing

344. In comparing alcohol consumption in women and men, each of the following is true EXCEPT that

(A) women and men who are heavy drinkers are equally susceptible to alcohol-related morbidity and mortality
(B) at comparable levels of alcoholism, alcoholic women would pose a greater cost to society
(C) in mixed company, women drink less
(D) the amount of alcoholism among men is greater
(E) social norms display less tolerance of heavy drinking in women

345. The World Health Organization has stated that the most serious worldwide drug problem is use of

(A) cocaine
(B) alcohol
(C) marijuana
(D) amphetamines
(E) opium

346. Persons of lower socioeconomic status (SES) have higher rates of all the following EXCEPT

(A) iatrogenic illness
(B) chronic illness
(C) obesity
(D) hypertension
(E) coronary artery disease

347. Rights and obligations of the sick role include all the following EXCEPT

(A) attempt to secure professional help
(B) ability to pay for treatment
(C) compliance with the prescribed regimen
(D) release from certain normal role obligations
(E) freedom from blame for being ill

348. All the following statements about persons of lower socioeconomic status (SES) and their attitudes toward health are true EXCEPT

(A) their medical needs are greater
(B) they are less concerned about their health
(C) they have a chronically low utilization rate of health services
(D) their health-seeking behaviors do not change even when financial barriers are removed
(E) they are more alienated from society and medical institutions

349. All the following stages of dying were elucidated by Kubler-Ross EXCEPT

(A) denial
(B) anger
(C) rejection of God or supreme being
(D) bargaining
(E) depression

350. Patients who are ill and facing death are LEAST likely to exhibit reactions to the loss of

(A) independence
(B) appetite
(C) self-image
(D) control
(E) financial resources

351. The factor that has the LEAST influence on the outcome of teenage pregnancy is

(A) maternal intake of protein calories
(B) maternal age at conception
(C) maternal educational level
(D) prenatal medical care
(E) paternal identity

352. Persons of low socioeconomic status (SES) are more apt to display all the following sick role behaviors or outcomes EXCEPT

(A) more self-medication
(B) more interest in medical care when ill
(C) longer hospital stays
(D) greater responsiveness to crises than to future objectives
(E) increased mortality from cancer once it occurs

DIRECTIONS: Each group of questions below consists of lettered headings followed by a set of numbered items. For each numbered item select the **one** lettered heading with which it is **most** closely associated. Each lettered heading may be used **once, more than once, or not at all.**

Questions 353–356

For each of the descriptions below, match the appropriate term.

(A) Authoritarian personality
(B) Discrimination
(C) Ethnic group
(D) Prejudice
(E) Minority

353. A group distinguished on the basis of socially or culturally acquired lifeways

354. An attitude of aversion or hostility toward members of another group simply because they are members and presumed to have the same objectionable characteristics attributed to the group

355. Denial of power, privilege, or status to members of one group whose qualifications are equal to those of the dominant group

356. Rigid, conventional thinking, highly judgmental values, and a cynical and "fascist" mind-set

Questions 357–360

For each description below, match the most appropriate model or theory related to compliance.

(A) Defense mechanism model
(B) Health perception model
(C) Health opinion survey model
(D) Health belief model
(E) Naive health theory (common-sense model of illness)

357. Asserts that the patient connects an apparently unrelated symptom with a disorder and complies only when the symptom arises

358. Measures a patient's preferences for more or less active participation

359. Links denial to recovery

360. Ties recovery and rehabilitation to a patient's perception of his or her own health

Sociocultural Patterns of Behavior

Answers

309. The answer is D. *(Rosenthal, 2/e, pp 190–191.)* Following World War II, many social psychologists studied the causes of fascism and anti-Semitism. Theodore Adorno and coworkers developed the F-scale (for fascism), which they believed to be a measure of the authoritarian personality. Persons scoring high on the F-scale generally are very rigid in their thinking, very aware of status differences between themselves and others, highly deferential to superiors, very strict with subordinates, and generally prejudiced toward ethnic and minority groups. Such a person is seen as aligning with authority figures, protective in-groups, nationalism, and rigid moralism and to perceive most things in absolute terms.

310. The answer is B. *(Gatchel, 2/e, pp 114–116.)* Genetic factors alone cannot account for the high prevalence of hypertension among various racial, social, and cultural groups. Compared with that among whites, the prevalence of hypertension among blacks is significantly higher. Hypertension is more prevalent among poor American blacks, however, than among blacks of middle and upper classes.

311. The answer is D. *(Lindzey, 3/e, pp 858–859.)* While fearfulness, confusion, interpersonal conflict, and regression can generate stress that can have a direct effect on biologic responses, the loss of perceived control can take an even greater toll on the body. Excessive workload and job responsibility are stressful factors in terms of coronary risk, but they become even more powerful and biologically more destructive when they approach the limit of a person's capacity to control his or her own work. Whether the stress is from employment, unemployment, finance, family, disease, or other factors, the threat of loss or actual loss of control over one's being or activities appears to be the most devastating influence. Different people also have considerable variability in their responsiveness to a lack of or loss of control; this responsiveness then has a subsequent effect on their biologic processes.

312. The answer is B. *(Twaddle, 2/e, pp 175–176.)* *Curanderismo* is a Mexican-American conception of disease that identifies imbalances of heat and cold within the body as the major cause of disease or illness. Certain diseases are considered hot and others cold. Hot foods (e.g., rice, pork, beans, onions, beer, and goat's milk) are used to cure cold illnesses (e.g., measles and ear infections), and cold foods (e.g., lamb, corn, tortillas, peas, cow's milk, and oatmeal) are used to cure hot illnesses (e.g., bleeding and skin disorders). Foods and herbs are considered hot or cold on the basis of their relationship to hot and cold forces within the body, not according to actual temperature. *Curanderos* practice as soloists and are respected and valued because they reflect and reinforce the culture of the *barrio*—the community. They share the same value system, norms, and symbol systems. The healer is truly of the people. This cultural congruence between healer and patient produces a close healer-patient relationship of the type that is all too rare in Western scientific medicine.

313. The answer is D. *(Vander Zanden, 4/e, pp 213–215.)* Most sociologists consider a norm to be a shared expectation concerning the behavior of a group or a particular person in a particular role. If a norm is violated, some type of sanction or punishment generally will be imposed on the violator. Although average behavior may be considered "normal," it is not normative unless it meets shared expectations and is subject to enforcement.

314. The answer is A. *(Vander Zanden, 4/e, pp 468–470.)* Racial prejudice is often so thoroughly learned that it is extremely difficult to modify. However, the most effective means of reducing racial prejudice has been found to be interracial contact. Since most black-white prejudices are formed in the context of lack of contact, prevention and attitude change can best be accomplished by multiple opportunities for blacks and whites to get to know each other. It is also important to recognize that the interracial situation should consist of equality of black-white status, a need for cooperation, very few members with negative stereotypes about each other, intimacy of interaction, and antiprejudice social norms and expectations. Introducing black studies into elementary school curricula, improving the black image in the mass media, legislating against prejudiced behavior, campaigns to counteract stereotypes, and the use of psychotherapy in treating black-white confrontation have all been of assistance in reducing prejudice but have not proved as powerful as interracial contact. There is still considerable controversy as to whether legislating against prejudiced behavior is an even more effective method of reducing racial prejudices. The old adage "a person convinced against his will is of the same opinion" still has some validity, but legislating against prejudiced behavior also has much validity. Perhaps at the interpersonal level the interracial contact is most important, while legislating has more societal importance.

315. The answer is D. *(Rosen, pp 13–15.)* Persons who tend to focus more on feelings and bodily changes have been shown to be more likely to experience disturbing and distressing states. Self-awareness achieved through such acts as being aware of test results and receiving medical information or counseling is positively correlated to psychological and physical health. Introspectiveness, however, emerges as the strongest predictor of distress, overshadowing all other predictors.

316. The answer is B. *(Twaddle, 2/e, pp 131–132.)* Studies by Zborowski (1952, 1969) revealed that American Italians and Jews were much more likely to be open and vocal about their discomfort than were Americans of Irish or "Old American" descent (the classification "Old American" refers to persons having several generations of ancestors born in the United States). The Italians focused on the pain itself, whereas the Jews worried about what the pain portended for the future. The Irish seemed to deny the existence of the pain, whereas the "Old Americans" described the pain in detail in a detached and scientific manner. Pain was measured both by a person's subjective ratings of discomfort on a scale from 1 to 10 and by responses on a standardized questionnaire.

317. The answer is D. *(Twaddle, 2/e, p 132.)* There are no ethnic differences in threshold for the sensation of pain. The ethnic response to pain, however, is highly variable and is conditioned by cultural factors. The ethnic significance and traditions of emotionalism or stoicism regarding pain are major factors in accounting for this variable response to pain.

318. The answer is B. *(Isselbacher, 13/e, pp 8–10.)* Ethnic origin and race are major factors in certain diseases. Insulin-dependent diabetes mellitus is more frequent in whites than in African-Americans and is even less common in blacks born and living in Africa. Non-insulin-dependent diabetes is twice as high in African-Americans and Native Americans. The prevalence of hypertension in African-Americans is two to four times that in whites, especially among African-American women, with a parallel increase in end-stage renal disease. The mechanism is unclear at this point, but is thought to be related to selective survival, diet (sodium intake), social stress, occupational insecurity, and genetics. The higher prevalence of obesity is related to diet and socioeconomic status. The incidence and prevalence of tuberculosis is twice as high in African-Americans as in whites. Genetic factors may play a dominant role, in addition to economic deprivation, overcrowding, and poor nutrition. Stroke and coronary mortality are higher in African-Americans than in whites, a fact thought to be related to the higher prevalence of hypertension, diabetes, and obesity. Other diseases with significant ethnic and racial associations are osteoporosis (white women); cancer of the esophagus, stomach, pancreas, lung, cervix, and prostate (African-Americans); cirrhosis (Hispanics); and arthritis and connective tissue disorders (whites). These differences emphasize the importance of understanding demographic and ethnic factors.

319. The answer is E. *(Twaddle, 2/e, pp 179–180.)* Chinese-American medicine assumes that each person has a vital force. In each person's life force there is a conflict between yin and yang, the cold and hot forces, respectively. Many treatments are associated with restoration of the appropriate balance of yin and yang. Foods and herbals are most commonly used for this purpose.

320. The answer is E. *(Sierles, p 101.)* The health belief model is a value-expectancy theory about the use of health care. The model states that people will decide logically how to implement their own values about health. The health belief model uses six variables to predict who will and who will not seek health care: perception of their own susceptibility to illness, perception of the seriousness of the illness, the benefits of seeking care, the perceived costs of the care, cues that led to contemplating the risk, and motivation to maintain health. While the model does predict use of health care by those of higher SES, it assumes a person has the socioeconomic resources to carry out rational decisions. It also overemphasizes the extent to which humans make rational decisions and does not recognize that there are often real barriers to perception of susceptibility, understanding of consequences, and benefits of seeking care, especially among the poor, rural, and older population.

321. The answer is A. *(Sierles, pp 97–100.)* A disease is a condition evidenced by a clinical or a laboratory diagnosis and labeling. To a physician, the pathologic findings are the determining factors. To the patient, the experience of not feeling well is evidence of sickness, especially in the presence of symptoms such as pain, fatigue, or discomfort. On the other hand, when patients feel no symptoms in such conditions as hypertension, hypercholesterolemia, or premature ventricular contractions, they will be more apt to deny illness or resist the notion that they must be treated because they are ill. They can be diseased according to the physician's criteria but not ill. Unfortunately the medical model primarily considers a direct relationship between pathology and illness, which tends to exclude the role of human behavior.

322. The answer is A. *(Isselbacher, 13/e, pp 10–14.)* Socioeconomic status (SES) is a major factor in morbidity and mortality. While there have been marked improvements in life expectancy over the past 50 years, there is greater morbidity and mortality among individuals of lower SES than those of higher SES. While behavioral risk factors play a major role in disease etiology and subsequent morbidity and mortality, they do not entirely explain the differences in disease prevalence. Coronary artery disease, stroke, lung cancer, and hypertension are only a few of the diseases experienced more frequently in persons of lower SES. In addition to lower income, lack of education is also a prominent factor in increased morbidity and mortality. Physicians must understand that lower SES influences the etiology and prognosis of disease through greater environmental exposure to toxins, an increase in behavioral risk factors, less access to health care, and less compliance with recommended regimens, among other factors.

323.   The answer is B. *(Schuster, 3/e, pp 296–297.)* There are many misconceptions regarding gender-related differences, often to justify role stereotyping. Some gender-related differences have been established through empirical research in the U.S. Females have greater verbal ability, while males have better visual-spatial skills, excel in mathematical skills, and are more aggressive. Also, females are generally more sensitive to sensory input and six times more likely to sing in tune, while males show greater field-independence of visual stimuli and are more sensitive to light. It is important to recognize that these are normative data and that there is much cross-over and overlap in normal development. Also, persons with a dynamic, flexible orientation toward life make the most positive adjustments to life. The interaction of sociocultural learning and individual biologic activity plays a major role in the development of gender-related differences.

324.   The answer is B. *(Twaddle, 2/e, pp 172–174.)* Most spiritual healers consider disease to be a result of psychological conflicts. Stress produced by this conflict ultimately yields symptoms that are identified as a disease entity. Healers believe that the conflict and stress will be relieved once affected patients submit to the larger plan of God. Some spiritual healers explain disease as the result of original sin or the disenchantment of heavenly spirits. The parapsychological perspective speculates that there is a radical interchange of energy between body, mind, and the psychoid or Jungian collective unconscious. The healing process involves a large-scale exchange of energy and equates an emotionally charged atmosphere with energy transfer and rapid resolution of illness. Some healers recognize a germ-mechanical theory of disease in which germs cause a deterioration of physical systems and recommend that patients seek resolution of the germ problem before spiritual healing can succeed. Few spiritual healers subscribe to the notion that disease results from the invasion of the body by evil spirits.

325.   The answer is A. *(Gatchel, 2/e, pp 172–173.)* The interpretation and reporting of symptoms is influenced by complex psychosocial and cultural factors. Studies comparing men and women in terms of their reporting of symptoms and their seeking help have found that women are more likely to report symptoms and to seek medical attention for them. Also, women are more accurate in reporting their symptoms. Persons of lower socioeconomic status are also more likely to report symptoms. Whether one seeks help is even more complex and depends on several intervening factors such as prior medical or psychological history, distress, social support, and economic factors.

326. The answer is A. *(Hamburg, pp 132–136.)* Malnutrition plays a major role in pregnancy at any age; it can be even more important, however, for a pregnant teenager, who is still growing and developing at the same time as the fetus. There are areas in all parts of the U.S. where pregnant teenagers, as well as other adolescents and children, are subjected to significant malnutrition and undernutrition. Protein-energy malnutrition and iodine and iron deficiencies are major health concerns. Socioeconomic and political factors, life-style, and ignorance play important roles. Studies of nutrition and weight gain during pregnancy have shown a strong relationship between the weight gain of pregnancy and infant birth weight. Mothers who were initially underweight and who gained less than 7 kg during pregnancy had a 40 percent risk of delivering a child of lower birth weight. Adolescent mothers had a greater risk of delivering an infant of low birth weight, and adolescents between 10 and 16 years of age delivered infants who were even more retarded in growth than those of older adolescents. Also, pregnant adolescents retain nitrogen less efficiently than do pregnant adult women.

327. The answer is A. *(U.S. Public Health Service, pp 1, 18, 88.)* Infant mortality in the U.S. is now about one-third the rate it was in 1950 (29.2 per 1000 births in 1950 versus 8.9 in 1991). Infant mortality for both black and white births in the U.S. has decreased at about the same rate since 1950, but black infant mortality remains more than twice as high as that for white infants (17.6 versus 7.3). Internationally, the U.S. ranks twenty-fourth among all countries. Japan has the lowest infant mortality of all countries (4.6 deaths per 1000 births) and is followed by Finland, Sweden, Hong Kong, Singapore, Canada, Switzerland, Germany, Norway, and the Netherlands. Canada ranks sixth among all nations. Availability and quality of prenatal and neonatal care are obviously major factors in comparing these countries with the United States.

328. The answer is E. *(Isselbacher, 13/e, pp 14–15.)* In the 1930s over 50 percent of men smoked versus only 20 percent of women. By 1960 about 50 percent of men still smoked, while the rate for women had risen to over 30 percent. By 1990 the rate for men had decreased to less than 30 percent and the rate for women had only decreased to about 25 percent. Thus, between

1960 and 1990 the rate of regular smokers decreased significantly for men, but much less for women. The cardiovascular mortality for men has decreased, and the lung cancer mortality for men has also begun to decrease. From 1960 to 1990, the mortality for lung cancer in women continued to increase so that it now exceeds the mortality for breast cancer and will probably continue to increase for a few years because the pattern of regular smoking (and lung cancer) for women appears to be following about 20 years behind the pattern for men. Even though "low-yield" cigarettes have been heavily marketed to women, the myocardial risk for low-yield versus higher yield cigarettes is the same. Behavioral change and educational strategies different from those for men should be explored for women.

329. The answer is A. *(Sierles, pp 345–346.)* During the 1980s all states passed legislation that was more effective in reducing vehicular accidents than were other strategies. The legislation involved stricter penalties for alcohol-impaired driving, mandatory participation in rehabilitation, establishment of illegal blood alcohol concentrations for drivers, and an increase in the legal drinking age to 21 years in all states. The effectiveness of legislation was increased by other preventive strategies, e.g., education, behavioral change, safety engineering, new technologies, and government safety standards. Seat belts and child restraint laws have reduced both injury and death in children and adults. States that raised their speed limit from 55 to 65 mph on rural interstates have experienced an increase in fatalities averaging 22 percent. In 1990 there were still 46,000 deaths and 2 million injuries from motor vehicle accidents.

330. The answer is D. *(Hamburg, pp 136–138.)* With the social and biologic trends of earlier menarche, reproductive readiness, and postponed adult roles, the median age for the initiation of sexual activity has dropped from 18 to 16 years. With such social changes as those in female roles, permissive attitudes, legalization of abortion, and change of traditional family patterns, the sexual behavior of adolescents has also changed. Even though the technology and availability of contraceptives have improved, the youngest of the adolescents are less likely than older women to use contraceptives. The abortion rate increased steadily from the Supreme Court decision in 1973 until about 1979, when it began to level off. Of the approximately 1 million adolescent pregnancies each year (which has increased recently), about 400,000 (40 percent) end in abortions. Contrary to conventional opinion, it has been found that an adolescent who has had an abortion is less likely to become pregnant again within 2 years than one who has given birth. Parental involvement in a teenager's abortion does not appear to reduce the probability of subsequent unwanted pregnancies.

331. The answer is D. *(Hazzard, 3/e, pp 126–133.)* Promoting healthy life-styles has been more effective in the most educated and older groups and less effective in less well educated and lower socioeconomic groups. Poverty also increases the incidence and prevalence of disease. It is significant that Social Security policy in the United States over the past 2 decades has reduced poverty among older adults, thus helping to reduce their vulnerability to disease. Social Security has been less successful for older unmarried women, however, as in 1984, 20 percent of them were still in poverty. In fact, women are two and a half times more likely than men to be poor or near poor. The differential life expectancy between lower and middle classes at birth is 5 years, but by the time they are elderly, the middle-class advantage has expanded to 9 years. The differential for disability-free years is over 13 years.

332. The answer is C. *(Rosen, pp 201–214.)* A person's beliefs are important determinants of preventive health behavior. Even though most patients with hypertension cannot determine when their blood pressure is abnormal, the majority believe they can. They are also more apt to believe that their own reading of symptoms and the fact of feeling better are more valid than their physician's instructions or reassurances. As a result, many patients will stop or change treatment on the basis of their feelings and symptoms. If patients have the belief that they can control their health outcome, they are more apt to try to be more successful in changing such health behaviors as smoking, diet, and exercise to prevent or to cure an illness. Older patients are more apt to believe that they can enhance their health by controlling their emotions (anger, anxiety, and depression) and staying mentally active. Younger people place more value on vigorous exercise to promote health and prevent illness.

333. The answer is A. *(Hazzard, 3/e, pp 125–129, 183–184.)* The maintenance of social connections and support has an important association with health and well-being throughout the life span. When compared with younger populations, however, elderly people are more apt to experience significant life changes such as death of a spouse and involuntary relocation. Also, the relative importance of specific social relationships may be different in the elderly. For example, marriage decreases the risk of mortality in younger populations, but seems to be less of a protective factor in older populations. Marital status is not a major predictor of mortality in the elderly because not having a spouse is a more normative experience and therefore is considered to be less stressful. The support of friends and other relatives becomes a more powerful predictor of mortality in the elderly group than in younger groups. Older groups are also less likely to maintain extensive contacts with multiple sources and will have more limited networks for support.

334. The answer is C. *(Sierles, pp 359–360.)* Those most prone to violence are male, young, and poor. Poverty is also overrepresented among victims of homicide, and women who are poor are more likely to be raped or attacked than other women. Other factors related to poverty—minimal education, poor health, family instability, and overcrowded and inadequate housing—are all highly associated with violence. While the age-adjusted homicide rates for some races are higher than others, race itself is not considered to be a major etiologic factor.

335. The answer is A. *(Sierles, pp 358–360.)* The vast majority of homicides are intraracial rather than interracial. In other words, Asian-Americans tend to kill Asian-Americans, Euro-Americans tend to kill Euro-Americans, and African-Americans tend to kill African-Americans. The most common homicide committed in the United States is by an acquaintance and is usually over a love triangle, money, or property. Males are nine times as likely to commit violent crimes, but the rate of violent crimes for females is increasing.

336. The answer is B. *(Sierles, pp 350–351.)* There are between 25,000 and 29,000 completed suicides in the United States each year and about 250,000 to 290,000 attempted suicides. The overall rate of suicide has changed very little since 1900. It tends to increase with age, but in the second half of this century, adolescent rates have increased tremendously, and for persons 50 years old, the rate has declined by almost as much. Suicide is the second leading cause of death for those 15 to 24 years old. Epidemiologists have found that media publicity about suicides, real or fictional, has a contagious effect, especially with adolescents. Males commit (complete) suicide 2 to 3 times as often as females and Euro-Americans commit suicide 2 to 3 times as often as African-Americans. At least 10 percent of persons who attempt suicide eventually are successful in killing themselves. In spite of conventional wisdom, poor persons do not have higher suicide rates than the economically privileged.

337. The answer is A. *(Isselbacher 13/e, pp 2420–2425.)* One of the most important aspects of identifying a person with a problem of alcoholism is to do an adequate social history. If the patient is having problems on the job, marital difficulties (which could also be with other members of the family), certain patterns of accidents, and driving-related difficulties, these can be considered behavioral markers for suspicion of excess drinking. There is a simple 25-item form (the Michigan Alcohol Screening Test, MAST) to be answered by the patient that explores other behaviorally related areas and is of great help in identifying the patient with alcohol-related problems. Often, the patient's complaints, such as insomnia or hypertension, can serve as a way of beginning to gain the patient's collaboration to do something about the alcohol problem. Other findings, such as multiple bouts of pneumonia, unexplained cardiac arrhythmias, cirrhosis, and pancreatitis, can also raise suspicions.

338. The answer is A. *(Rosen, pp 97–98.)* Dieting induced by social and cultural pressures initiates a process of biologic, cognitive, and behavioral disregulation. The first effect of reducing the intake of calories is a lowered basal metabolic rate, which does not immediately increase after the dieting has ceased; this results in a net increase in calories and weight. Also, hormonal changes occur after dieting, especially after severe dieting, that actually promote fat storage. Other biologic changes induced by dieting include plateaus in weight loss, cravings, or binges, and the frequent development of increasingly compulsive strategies in attempts to lose weight. These mechanisms can actually result in weight gain, especially over the long term, since external pressures are generally not effective for maintenance of weight loss.

339. The answer is D. *(Conger, 4/e, pp 428–430.)* College students who do not drink alcohol tend to come from rural, conservative, and deeply religious (usually Protestant) backgrounds. Heavy use of alcohol is found more frequently among social science majors from metropolitan areas, particularly those who are pessimistic about their future. Heavy drinkers are more likely than nondrinkers to use nonalcoholic drugs and have a higher rate of academic failure and drop-out. Their parents are more likely to drink, as well as their friends and best friends.

340. The answer is C. *(Linden, pp 22–24.)* Many Asians exhibit a general flushing response to the ingestion of alcohol. This aversive effect of alcohol has been attributed to genetics and results in an exaggerated sensitivity. They also have a lower rate of alcoholism than do Caucasians. Asians and Caucasians do not differ in the oxidation rate of alcohol. Many Asians, however, develop higher levels of acetylaldehyde after consumption. Japanese subjects, in particular, have been shown to develop an atypical form of alcohol dehydrogenase (ADH) enzyme that more rapidly produces acetylaldehyde, resulting in higher levels of accumulation. This particular allele is found in 85 percent of Asians and only 6 percent of Europeans. Many Asians have demonstrated a stronger reactivity in heart rate. Blood pressure, as well as facial flushing, is also increased to a greater extent than in Caucasians. And Asians report that they experience more subjective discomfort following alcohol consumption than do Caucasians.

341. The answer is E. *(Rosen, pp 46–49.)* Alcoholism among both male and female homosexuals is estimated to be between 20 and 32 percent. Although there is considerable variation among races and nationalities, Asian Americans tend to drink less alcohol than non-Asian Americans. They also metabolize ethanol more quickly. Rates of alcoholism among Hispanic Americans appear to be higher than the national average and are thought to be related to sociocultural norms and values. Alcoholism among American Indians and native Alaskans is high, and the rate of alcoholism becomes even higher when American Indians from reservations enter the urban environment. Alcoholism among blacks appears to be increasing with little recognition of its threat. In terms of prevention, all minority groups suffer from a lack of targeted treatment and prevention programs; they also tend not to use the few existing programs.

342. The answer is B. *(Hazzard, 3/e, pp 125–150.)* The number of persons over the age of 65 has continued to increase in this century from 3.1 million in 1900 to 24.1 million in 1978. The proportion of the over-65 age group also rose from 4.1 percent to 11 percent. By the year 2000, the over-65 age group was expected to increase to 32 million and 12 percent of the population, but present declining mortality could result in 38 million and about 14 percent of the total population by the year 2000. In 1978, the over-75 age group was 38 percent of the total over-65 age group, and it is estimated that by 2003 the over-75 age group will have increased to about 47 percent. Thus more of the population has been reaching the 65-and-older age group, and living longer, and will continue to do so. Also, among the elderly the female population has progressively outnumbered the male population. The 80 men per 100 women in the 65-to-69-year-old group decreases to 45 men per 100 women in the 85-and-over population. While the 80 men per 100 women in the 65-to-69-year-old group is expected to rise slightly to 82 by the year 2000 and 83 by 2020, the men per 100 women in the 85-and-over group is expected to fall to 39 in 2000 and slightly below 39 by 2020. Only about 5 percent of the over-65 age group are in institutions (e.g., long-term facilities and nursing homes), which means that about 95 percent of the elderly are attempting to live with some measure of independence. A disproportional number of the institutionalized elderly are white (94 percent), and there are twice as many females as males.

343. The answer is D. *(Twaddle, 2/e, p 178.)* In contrast to Western scientific medicine, practitioners of Native-American medicine never considered blood-letting to be of medical value. They have employed a wide variety of drugs, however, such as astringents, emetics, sedatives, stimulants, antibiotics, and even pharmacologic contraceptives. Mechanical treatments have included quarantine, sweat baths, bathing in mineral springs, surgery, and immobilization of broken limbs. Spiritual methods employed in Native-American medicine and carried out by a shaman include group singing, incantations, and facilitation of communication with the spirits by smoking the peace pipe.

344. The answer is A. *(Rosen, pp 38–41.)* Scandinavian, Canadian, and American studies comparing the alcohol drinking patterns of women with those of men show that women have significantly higher morbidity and mortality as a result of alcohol consumption. For example, they are more successful with suicide and more apt to die from both accidents and cirrhosis of the liver. The more toxic effect of alcohol on the hypothalamic-pituitary-gonadal axis in women and genetic predispositions are thought to be prominent factors. Women are known to drink less than men in general, and even less in mixed company. The overall severity of alcoholism in women is less than in men. Some of this is attributed to the fact that social norms are less tolerant of heavy drinking in women. Because of the effects of alcohol on such factors as fertility, miscarriage, cirrhosis, suicide, and sexual dysfunction, the cost to society of comparable levels of alcoholism appears to be even greater for women than men.

345. The answer is B. *(Hamburg, p 207.)* Alcohol use and abuse is thought to be the most serious worldwide drug problem. It affects many millions of adult problem drinkers, as well as their families, friends, coworkers, and innocent victims of alcohol-related accidents and violence. About 50 percent of motor vehicle deaths are related to alcohol and it is estimated that about 10 percent of all deaths in developed nations are the result of misuse of alcohol. It is also a causal factor in damage to the liver and brain and is involved in some cancers. Cocaine, opium, marijuana, and amphetamines are major problems in the world, but they tend to be more localized in certain regions or cultures, whereas alcohol use is ubiquitous.

346. The answer is A. *(Sierles, pp 94–97.)* The most powerful biopsychosocial predictor of prevalence of illness, morbidity, and mortality is socioeconomic status (SES). Persons of lower SES have a significantly higher prevalence of obesity, chronic illnesses, hypertension, and coronary artery disease. This can be attributed to multiple factors, including lack of access to medical care, lack of resources to seek medical care, living and working in a high-risk environment, dietary deficiencies, lack of educational background, lack of responsiveness of physicians to patients of lower SES and their problems, and the general lack of societal and political concern with the health of the poor. Iatrogenic illness is not as frequent in persons of lower SES because they have less contact with the remedies of physicians and medical technology.

347. The answer is B. *(Sierles, pp 99–101.)* In order to enter a sick role, the patients must be willing and able to seek professional help for their symptoms, comply with the prescribed regimen, accept release from their normal role obligations, and be considered as blameless for their illness. The sick role bears no relation to the ability or willingness to pay for treatment. The blamelessness and the relaxed role obligations are considered rights, while the seeking of professional help and the willingness to comply with a prescribed treatment are considered obligations. The sick role is now being challenged somewhat by changing cultural values that encourage (sometimes insist) people to accept responsibility for their own health, e.g., by avoiding smoking, obesity, or HIV infection to the extent possible.

348. The answer is B. *(Last, 13/e, pp 638–639.)* People of lower income have a chronically low rate of utilization of medical care facilities. They have a greater need for medical care and are more concerned about their health, yet they exhibit greater tolerance for or endurance of symptoms. The lower rates of utilization are often explained on the basis of the inadequate financial resources; the "culture of poverty," in which the poor are more apt to be alienated from society and medical institutions; and the barriers that the poor encounter, such as the greater distances from medical care facilities, the longer waits and impersonal care, the fragmented services, and a lack of understanding of how to use the system. An interesting finding is that the provision of financial assistance packages and improved access to prepaid programs does not significantly change the health-seeking behavior patterns. This would suggest the role of certain social, psychological, and cultural factors in the problem.

349. The answer is C. *(Sierles, pp 169–170.)* Kubler-Ross identified five psychological stages of dying or facing the death of a loved one. The first stage is denial or disbelief about the diagnosis or the fatal prognosis. Next is anger expressed at oneself, the doctors, God, or whomever one holds responsible. Bargaining (usually with God) follows, such as promising better behavior in the hopes of survival. Depression often follows until acceptance is achieved. It is important to recognize that, just as with stages of normal development, there is much overlap between each stage, and "recycling" of unresolved portions of different stages occurs until acceptance or an acceptable level of coping occurs.

350. The answer is B. *(Hazzard, 3/e, pp 383–390.)* Patients facing the threat of death most often exhibit physical and emotional reactions to loss. The most frequent losses are of independence, self-image, control, and financial security. The loss of independence is particularly upsetting to persons who have always taken care of their own physical needs but who now need help with simple daily tasks. The dependency generated by intense pain is of great concern to dying patients. Earning power, mobility, and family or job role are also important parts of independence. Loss of self-image through change of personal appearance, weakness, disfigurement, and embarrassingly altered body function is also disturbing. Loss of control is one of the most upsetting conflicts and often results from the control and authority assumed by the medical profession. Patients often fear that they will be abandoned if they do not relinquish complete control over their lives. The loss of financial resources engendered by illness, e.g., the threat of financial hardship or loss of one's entire life savings, is also of major concern for the dying patient. Dying patients usually are not hungry and do not express concern for food.

351. The answer is E. *(Hamburg, pp 134–136.)* It is now known that the intake of protein calories is a major determinant of the outcome of teenage pregnancy, yet many pregnant adolescents are malnourished in this regard and produce an increasing incidence of low–birth-weight babies and fetal wastage. The younger the age at conception, especially for mothers under 16 years of age, the greater the number and severity of risk factors. Postnatal medical care is important, but prenatal care has been demonstrated to be even more crucial. This is especially true from the standpoint of prevention of some risk factors that can be modified or averted. Adolescent pregnancy is positively linked to low educational status in that education is often interrupted or terminated, which significantly reduces the life options of the adolescent mother and results in low-paying jobs throughout adult life. The result is most often a single-parent household, stress, and greatly reduced educational and psychological growth. These socioeconomic and behavioral factors can result in outcomes for both the pregnant adolescent and the developing child more destructive than the potential physical and biomedical problems. The children of adolescent mothers have a higher percentage of developmental, behavioral, and cognitive difficulties than children of older mothers. While the identity of the father could play a role in terms of identifying genetic factors, transmission of sexually transmitted diseases, and potential source of marriage and support, it is not as important a factor as nutrition, age, educational potential, or prenatal care.

352. The answer is B. *(Sierles, pp 94–97.)* Socioeconomic status (SES) is a powerful predictor of individual sick role behavior. Studies have documented that persons of low SES use more self-medication, stay in the hospital for a longer period of time, have a greater responsiveness to crises than to future objectives, planning, or chronic conditions, and are more apt to die from cancer once it occurs. They also have less interest in medical care when they are ill, are more apt to see nonmedical personnel for treatment, and demonstrate less adherence to schedules.

353–356. The answers are 353-C, 354-D, 355-B, 356-A. *(Vander Zanden, 4/e, pp 409, 460–465, 467–471, 490.)* An ethnic group is a group distinguished on the basis of socially acquired lifeways. The members are usually biologically related and are related on the basis of common customs or culture (e.g., Italian or Irish).

Prejudice is described as a hostile or aversive attitude toward the members of a group simply because they belong to it and are therefore presumed to have the same objectionable qualities attributed to the group. The basic factors that characterize prejudice in the dominant group are feelings of superiority; the perception that the minority group is inherently different and alien; a claim to power, privilege, or status; and a fear or suspicion that the minority group wants the power, privilege, or status of the dominant group. Also, prejudice has a cognitive component (mental image), an affective component (feelings or emotions), and a behavioral component (predisposition to act).

Discrimination is an arbitrary denial of power, privilege, or status to a group (usually a minority) whose qualifications are equal to those of the dominant group. It is important to note that prejudice may or may not be associated with discrimination.

The authoritarian personality is characterized by rigid and conventional thinking, obsession with power and submission to authority, and highly judgmental values. T. W. Adorno characterized the authoritarian personality as having a mind-set similar to that of a fascist. There does appear to be a link between prejudice and authoritarianism.

A minority group is any racial or ethnic group that has hereditary membership, a consciousness of oneness, and a high degree of in-group marriage and usually suffers oppression from a dominant (majority) segment of a nation or state. The members often find themselves disadvantaged in terms of privilege and status, and the minority is often the source of dominant group's advantages.

357–360. The answers are 357-E, 358-C, 359-A, 360-B. *(Gatchel, 2/e, pp 174–196.)* The *health belief model* is useful in predicting compliance. Patients' perception of the severity of their condition and the extent to which they perceive themselves as being susceptible play a major role in whether or to what extent they will act to comply with the treatment regimen. Other factors to be assessed are patients' perceptions of the costs and benefits of compliance. The physician can use the beliefs and perceptions of patients to assist in the communication process and to predict when the patient is more apt to follow the recommended treatment.

The *naive health theory* proposed by Leventhal (also called the common-sense model of illness) asserts that many patients identify a medically unrelated symptom as being related to their disorder and they often limit their compliance to the presence of the unrelated symptom. An example would be a patient with hypertension who identifies the occurrence of a headache with the state of the hypertension. Even though objective evidence indicates that patients cannot reliably identify or predict changes in their blood pressure, the naive causal connection is made between the headaches and the blood pressure. The connection is reinforced when the patient develops a headache, measures his or her blood pressure, and indeed sees that it is elevated. The patient then reduces compliance to instances when a headache develops.

The *health opinion survey* measures patients' preferences for more or less active participation in their own health care and their preferences for a more or less informed role. Compliance is related to the degree of involvement and amount of information a patient prefers. Knowledge of these preferences allows the physician to attempt to match patients with the best treatment intervention to enhance compliance.

The *defense mechanism model* links a patient's own psychological defense mechanisms with compliance and recovery. Denial is a particularly important defense mechanism that is often used by the coronary patient. Since denial reduces stress, coronary patients who use denial in the critical care unit will experience less anxiety than those who do not. The moderate use of denial in the early phases of a myocardial infarction has been found to enhance recovery and survival. Those who use denial to an excessive extent, however, can actually endanger their recovery because they are less apt to comply with medical recommendations.

The *health perception model* is based on how patients view the status of their own health or illness. Patients who perceive their health to be poor have lower morale and are less likely to recover as rapidly and to return to work or to their normal activities than are those who perceive their health as relatively good and have an optimistic view of their health. These perceptions of one's health affect compliance and suggest several interventions that can be used to modify patients' perceptions of their health, such as education, instruction, nursing care, brief psychotherapy, and other means of encouraging as realistic and optimistic a view of recovery as possible.

Human Ecology and Disease

DIRECTIONS: Each question below contains five suggested responses. Select the **one best** response to each question.

361. Hospital patients who are well behaved but experience a state of helplessness are

(A) more likely to try to improve their own condition
(B) less apt to withhold information
(C) apt to be more informed about their own condition
(D) invariably happy to leave the hospital
(E) less able to accomplish the transition back to normal life after leaving the hospital

362. By the year 2000 the World Health Organization (WHO) is predicting that

(A) 20 million people will be infected with HIV
(B) 5 million people will have AIDS
(C) AIDS will kill 250,000 children under 5 years of age each year in central and east Africa
(D) 1 to 2 million children will be orphans from AIDS parents in central and east Africa
(E) AIDS will have penetrated at least two-thirds of the 162 countries of the world

363. Which of the following statements best describes the incidence, prevalence, or mortality of AIDS at the end of 1991 in the United States?

(A) From 1988 to 1991 AIDS increased from the fifteenth to the ninth leading cause of death
(B) Five percent of the AIDS cases have occurred in children under 13 years of age
(C) Twenty percent of AIDS cases have occurred in Euro-Americans
(D) By 1991 AIDS had killed almost as many Americans as the 55,000 Americans who were killed in the Vietnam War
(E) AIDS cases in women are now increasing at the same rate as men

364. Which of the following countries has the lowest prevalence of HIV/AIDS infection?

(A) Canada
(B) Cuba
(C) Netherlands
(D) Norway
(E) Sweden

365. Which of the following had the greatest change in prevalence over the past decade?

(A) Obesity
(B) Cigarette smoking for college graduates
(C) Tuberculosis
(D) Out-of-wedlock births
(E) Lack of insurance for medical care

366. The incidence of smoking addiction among high school seniors

(A) is more influenced by caring adults than by peer pressure
(B) can be reduced significantly by caring adults
(C) can be reduced significantly through arousal of fear
(D) exceeds the level of the general adult population
(E) occurs in an upward trend from elementary and junior high school

367. Over the past decade, which one of the following had the greatest increase?

(A) Pregnancy rate for teenagers
(B) Poverty rate for children under age 18
(C) Infants born weighing less than 2500 g
(D) Mortality for chronic obstructive pulmonary disease
(E) Mortality for lung cancer

368. Over the past decade, which one of the following showed the greatest decrease in mortality?

(A) Diseases of the heart
(B) Cerebrovascular diseases
(C) Breast cancer
(D) Unintentional injuries
(E) Motor vehicle crashes

369. Lung cancer is the most preventable cause of death in the United States. Which of the following is the second most preventable?

(A) Heart disease
(B) Cerebrovascular diseases
(C) Suicide
(D) Homicide
(E) Motor vehicle accidents

370. Which of the following social variables is most closely linked to infant mortality?

(A) Poverty
(B) Education of mother
(C) Education of father
(D) Occupation of father
(E) Marital status of parents

371. Compared with pregnant adult mothers, pregnant adolescent mothers have which of the following characteristics?

(A) Increased rates of toxemia
(B) Fewer placental abruptions
(C) Fewer infections of amniotic fluid
(D) Similar patterns of labor
(E) Similar amounts of cigarette and alcohol use

372. Which of the following causes a person to use the most calories per hour above basal metabolism?

(A) Bicycling (moderate speed)
(B) Walking (3 mph)
(C) Dancing (fox-trot)
(D) Swimming (2 mph)
(E) Horseback riding (trot)

373. True statements about alcohol abuse include that

(A) the percentage of families with problem-drinking men increases with age of head of household
(B) alcoholism is the second most frequent form of drug dependence after tobacco use in the United States
(C) the highest mortality from alcohol abuse is from accidents, followed by suicide and cirrhosis of the liver
(D) the annual cost to industry and the economy of alcohol abuse is currently estimated to be less than the cost of tobacco-related disease and death
(E) as a group, heavy drinkers of alcohol contribute more to national alcohol-related problems than does the group of moderate drinkers

374. During the first year after myocardial infarction, the majority of patients exhibit which of the following responses?

(A) Extensive disturbances in objective state
(B) Very little physical distress
(C) Perception of selves as not handicapped
(D) Depression and anxiety
(E) Perception of selves as having returned to normal

375. The fourth leading cause of death in early adolescence (10 to 14 years old) and the second leading cause of death in late adolescence and young adulthood is

(A) unintentional injury
(B) overdose of drugs or alcohol
(C) homicide
(D) suicide
(E) motor vehicle accidents

376. In the U.S., the leading cause of death among women is

(A) breast cancer
(B) lung cancer
(C) motor vehicle accidents
(D) cerebrovascular disease
(E) ischemic heart disease

377. The fastest growing age group in the United States is

(A) adolescents
(B) young adults
(C) middle-aged persons
(D) persons 65 to 79 years of age
(E) persons 80 years of age and older

378. When a "code" call for cardiopulmonary resuscitation (CPR) occurs on a general hospital service, the chance that the patient will survive to discharge is about

(A) 5 percent
(B) 10 percent
(C) 15 percent
(D) 20 percent
(E) 25 percent

379. The most common cause of dementia in the United States is

(A) infectious (viral or bacterial) dementia
(B) multi-infarct dementia
(C) Alzheimer's disease
(D) dementia with basal ganglia disease
(E) dementia with psychiatric disorders

380. The leading cause of death in the elderly (age 65 and older) is

(A) cancer
(B) cerebrovascular disease (stroke)
(C) suicide
(D) heart disease
(E) chronic obstructive pulmonary disease

DIRECTIONS: Each numbered question or incomplete statement below is NEGATIVELY phrased. Select the **one best** lettered response.

381. Obesity has been well documented as a primary contributing factor in the development of each of the following diseases EXCEPT

(A) adult-onset diabetes
(B) hypertension
(C) gallbladder disease
(D) arthritis
(E) myocardial hypertrophy

382. Behavioral research on nutrition and obesity has demonstrated that all the following are true EXCEPT

(A) eating is often a response to, compensation for, or defense against tension and frustration
(B) analyzing conditions under which one usually eats facilitates weight control
(C) psychological makeup influences eating behaviors and activity levels
(D) there are consistent, identifiable personality factors common to persons who have difficulty making a satisfactory weight adjustment
(E) weight gain occurs when energy intake exceeds energy output

383. Changes in life-style had caused a decline in each of the following diseases before the application of modern medicine and technology EXCEPT

(A) tuberculosis
(B) prostatic carcinoma
(C) rheumatic heart disease
(D) coronary artery disease
(E) stroke

384. Behavioral medicine has demonstrated significant contributions to the treatment of all the following diseases or conditions EXCEPT

(A) hypertension
(B) cardiac arrhythmias
(C) Raynaud's disease
(D) third-degree heart block
(E) asthma

385. The food aversion paradigm is involved in medicine in all the following EXCEPT

(A) chronic alcoholism
(B) chronic pain
(C) Addison's disease
(D) cancer
(E) chemotherapy

386. Which of the following markers is the LEAST effective predictor of morbidity and longevity?

(A) Gender
(B) Income
(C) Psychological markers
(D) Age
(E) Marital status

387. All the following statements concerning the mechanisms of the development of coronary heart disease are currently held to be true EXCEPT that

(A) repeated excessive heart rate or pressor responses to behavioral stressors can promote arterial injury through turbulence and sheer stress
(B) increased output of catecholamines and corticosteroids is biochemically toxic to coronary arteries
(C) increased circulating catecholamines influence platelet aggregation and the mobilization of serum lipids
(D) acute behavioral stressors can raise thresholds for ventricular fibrillation
(E) disruption of central nervous system control of the heart can initiate arrhythmic activity

388. All the following statements about teenage smoking are true EXCEPT that

(A) the age for beginning smoking is decreasing
(B) the majority of female smokers begin smoking after they are 13 years of age
(C) 12 percent of those 12 to 17 years of age smoke
(D) 26 percent of those 17 to 18 years of age smoke
(E) one-third of all 18 year olds are regular smokers

389. Active versus inactive persons usually report all the following psychological factors EXCEPT

(A) less depression
(B) less anxiety
(C) less type A behavior
(D) more hostility
(E) more self-confidence

390. Use of drugs by the elderly can be characterized by all the following statements EXCEPT

(A) over-the-counter medications account for 40 percent of drugs consumed
(B) psychotropic agents surpass all other drugs consumed by the institutionalized elderly
(C) over half of patients over age 60 make one or more medication errors during each illness
(D) a high risk factor for adverse drug reactions is being a male
(E) about 25 percent of national drug expenditures is consumed by the elderly

391. General characteristics of life events found to be very important in linking stress and illness include all the following EXCEPT

(A) desirability of an event
(B) reappraisal of a threat
(C) perceived control of an event
(D) effort required for readjustment
(E) frequency of an event

392. Each of the following statements about sleep problems is true EXCEPT that

(A) the number of people who have a sleep problem is about 50 percent
(B) pain and trouble sleeping are the two most common complaints in medicine
(C) insomnia is the chronic inability to obtain the necessary amount or quality of sleep to maintain adequate daytime behavior
(D) there is little evidence that sleeping medication is effective for more than several days
(E) there is an excessive tendency for poor sleepers to self-medicate and for physicians to over-prescribe strong sleeping pills

393. Studies of the links between psychological factors and disease states during and after World War II found all the following EXCEPT that

(A) blood pressure of Londoners increased during the initial phase of bombing
(B) survivors of concentration camps showed greater rates of physical illness
(C) survivors of concentration camps were better able to cope with cancer
(D) survivors of concentration camps showed a higher incidence of premature death following release
(E) survivors of concentration camps showed increased rates of relatively permanent problems of psychological adjustment

394. The following statements about alcohol and alcoholism are true EXCEPT that

(A) 10 percent of men and 3 to 5 percent of women develop alcoholism
(B) the homeless or skid-row alcoholic represents over 25 percent of all alcoholics
(C) there is considerable genetic variability controlling a person's response to alcohol
(D) 10 g of ethanol is equal to about 12 oz of beer, 4 oz of nonfortified wine, and 1.5 oz of 80-proof beverage
(E) alcoholics have a carcinoma rate 10 times higher than that of the general population

395. Anorexia nervosa involves concern about all the following EXCEPT

(A) body image
(B) control
(C) achievement
(D) sexuality
(E) dieting out of control

396. Patients with metastatic breast cancer are LEAST likely to live significantly longer if they are

(A) negatively reactive
(B) depressed
(C) married
(D) able to express hostility
(E) active in a social network

397. Empirical findings about patterns of disease and illness include all the following EXCEPT

(A) a large range of symptoms (e.g., headache, upset stomach, and sore muscles) is found in the general population on any given day
(B) a very small percentage of persons experiencing symptoms of disease or illness seeks medical care
(C) individual persons show highly diverse reactions to the presence of many disease symptoms
(D) it is important for physicians to understand how patients interpret their perceived physical signs and symptoms
(E) persons are relatively independent of communication from others in deciding on the meaning of their own unexpected physiologic changes

398. True statements about the placebo effect include all the following EXCEPT

(A) it is useful in the treatment of anxiety
(B) it involves β-endorphins
(C) it is useful in psychotherapy
(D) it is an important factor in biofeedback
(E) placebos have no effect when used in conjunction with chemically active drugs

399. All the following statements about hyperthyroidism are true EXCEPT that it

(A) may be the cause of a frank psychosis
(B) is more frequent in women than in men
(C) may be precipitated by acute emotional stress
(D) is associated with mental retardation in children
(E) is associated with tension and hyperexcitability

400. Behavioral prodromes of myocardial infarction and sudden death include all the following EXCEPT

(A) emotional exhaustion
(B) disregard of time pressures
(C) feelings of despair
(D) hopelessness
(E) depression

401. Adolescents represent about 17 percent of the population (40 million citizens), yet they account for all the following EXCEPT

(A) over twice as many automobile accidents as adults
(B) 20 percent of all suicides (5000 to 7000 adolescent suicides per year)
(C) over 600,000 pregnancies in unmarried girls per year
(D) the only age group for which the death rate is actually decreasing
(E) an age group of which over 12 percent smoke

402. Research studies support all the following findings about the health consequences of smoking behavior EXCEPT

(A) average life expectancy is decreased by 5 to 6 years
(B) most deaths caused by bronchitis/emphysema are smoking-related
(C) most deaths caused by lung cancer are smoking-related
(D) lung cancer deaths are actually decreasing for women
(E) most deaths caused by cancer of the oral cavity are smoking-related

403. The antidepressant effects of exercise have been linked with all the following EXCEPT

(A) increased cerebral blood flow
(B) increased levels of epinephrine and norepinephrine
(C) sense of mastery and self-control
(D) cathartic inhibition
(E) positive self-image

404. Studies of birth weight of human infants show all the following to be true EXCEPT

(A) black mothers give birth to small babies (2500 g or less) at a higher rate than do white mothers
(B) the most significant characteristic associated with a poor outcome of pregnancy is low birth weight
(C) babies of low birth weight, when compared with heavier babies, are likely to have a greater rate of developmental problems (epilepsy, cerebral palsy, mental retardation)
(D) the most frequently cited factors contributing to low birth weight are lack of prenatal care, poor nutrition, smoking, stress, and poor physical condition
(E) the geographic regions in the United States achieving lower-than-average birth weights in 1991 were New England and the Pacific region

405. Statistics on adolescent suicide show all the following patterns EXCEPT

(A) boys are three times more likely to commit suicide than are girls
(B) adolescents account for 6000 of the 28,000 suicides committed in the United States each year
(C) boys tend to choose more violent methods for committing suicide than do girls
(D) between 1970 and 1980, the suicide rate for teenage boys decreased
(E) schizophrenia may underlie the suicide

406. In a clinical setting, the diagnosis of alcoholism is made when a patient does all the following EXCEPT

(A) ignores early warning signs that alcohol is causing problems in marriage and moves ahead to separation or divorce
(B) is fired or laid-off as a result of alcohol-related problems
(C) demonstrates evidence of a preexisting antisocial personality disorder
(D) is arrested two or more times for an alcohol offense
(E) demonstrates signs of alcoholic withdrawal

DIRECTIONS: The group of questions below consists of lettered headings followed by a set of numbered items. For each numbered item select the **one** lettered heading with which it is **most** closely associated. Each lettered heading may be used **once, more than once, or not at all**.

Questions 407–410

For each condition, select the factor with which it is most significantly associated in the United States.

(A) Poverty
(B) Aging
(C) Heredity
(D) Religion
(E) Race

407. Sickle cell anemia

408. Phenylketonuria

409. Osteoarthritis

410. Dental decay

Human Ecology and Disease

Answers

361. The answer is E. *(Gatchel, 2/e, pp 163–165.)* Helplessness is based on the belief that one cannot meaningfully affect what happens. Thus, when hospitalized patients feel helpless, they are less likely to try to improve their own condition, they are less informed about their own condition, and they are more apt to withhold information that might even be helpful. As helplessness does generalize, they will be less able to feel that they can cope with the transition back to their normal life out of the hospital. They are often reluctant to leave the hospital, especially after an extended stay. Helplessness will also inhibit decision-making and such patients are often unwilling or unable to make decisions.

362. The answer is C. *(Sierles, pp 7–8.)* The World Health Organization (WHO) has declared that AIDS is an international epidemic. By the year 2000 it is predicted that there will be 40 million people infected with HIV and 10 million with active AIDS. WHO also expects that by the year 2000 in central and east Africa alone, AIDS will kill over 250,000 children each year under 5 years of age and that there will be 3 to 5 million orphans. Each of the 162 countries and six inhabited continents of the world has reported cases of AIDS.

363. The answer is A. *(Sierles, pp 7–8.)* AIDS cases have been reported in all 50 states with 83 percent of the cases in urban areas (500,000 population or more), 11 percent in cities of 50,000 to 500,000, and 6 percent in towns or rural areas of less than 50,000. From 1988 to 1991 AIDS increased from the fifteenth to the ninth leading cause of death. Two percent of the AIDS cases have been children under 13 years of age, and 10 percent of adolescents and adults with AIDS have been women. Fifty-four percent of AIDS cases have been in Euro-Americans, 20 percent in African-Americans, 16 percent in Hispanic-Americans, and 0.6 percent in Asian-Americans and Native Americans. By 1991 AIDS had already killed more than twice as many American men and women as the 55,000 Americans killed in the Vietnam War. The most common behavioral mode of transmission in America has been unprotected sex between men (65 percent). Sharing contaminated needles in drug injections accounted for 19 percent, and contaminated blood transfusions about 3 percent. AIDS cases in women are increasing at about twice the rate of men.

364. The answer is B. *(Sierles, p 11.)* HIV infection and AIDS is rare in Cuba (0.00009 percent of adult population). This is attributed to the fact that nearly everyone over 15 years of age has been tested for HIV and those who have tested positive (several hundred persons) have been quarantined and publically supported, similar to the way the U.S. used to quarantine persons infected with tuberculosis and leprosy. The Netherlands government encourages a program of voluntary information, condoms, and needle exchange among IV drug users, who have a prevalence of about 30 percent HIV infection. This has helped reduce the prevalence of HIV/AIDS, but has not controlled the infection. Canada, Norway, and Sweden have a significantly lower prevalence of HIV infection than the U.S., but like the U.S. they are not able to reduce or control the prevalence of HIV infection with voluntary programs.

365. The answer is D. *(U.S. Public Health Service, pp 1–8.)* The greatest change in prevalence over the past decade in the categories listed was in unmarried mothers. The increase in live births was 60 percent (95 percent increase in Euro-American mothers, compared with 41 percent in Native American mothers and 21 percent in African-American mothers). Overall, 29.5 percent of all live births are to unmarried mothers. The next greatest change was a 37 percent increase in persons under age 65 with no health insurance (an increase from 12.5 percent to 17.2 percent and still increasing). College graduates decreased their smoking by 35 percent, but persons with less than 12 years of education decreased only 10 percent. The current prevalence of smokers is 15 percent for college graduates and 37 percent for persons with less than a high school education. Overweight persons increased from 25 percent in 1970 to 33 percent in 1991; most of the increase occurred during the last decade. Tuberculosis, which was supposed to be all but eliminated, has shown a 20 percent increase over the past 5 years (27,000 cases). Part of this increase is due to increased prevalence as a coinfection with AIDS, but also among the homeless and prison inmates. The most rapid increase is due to new multiple-drug–resistant (MDR) strains with a mortality of 50 percent.

366. The answer is E. *(Rosen, pp 22–30.)* Peer pressure has been found to be more influential than any adult involvement in pre-adult smoking behavior. Even well-intentioned adults are often labeled as adult "naggers." Smoking often begins in elementary school, but most significantly in junior high school, and continues in an upward trend into high school, where by the senior year smoking addiction approaches the level of that in the general adult population. Arousal of fear has not been shown to be very effective in attempts to educate youth against smoking, alcohol use, or drug abuse.

367. The answer is D. *(U.S. Public Health Service, pp 1–3.)* In the past decade, mortality for chronic obstructive pulmonary diseases has increased 30 percent so that it now is the fourth leading cause of death in the United States. For women, the increase was more than 75 percent. The increase was relatively small for white males, but increased 24 percent for black males. For black males and females under 55 years of age, mortality was 2 to 5 times that for white males and females. Lung cancer mortality increased over 15 percent, but for women the increase was 45 percent. The rate of low birth weight (less than 2500 g) increased slightly from 6.8 to 7.1 percent of all live-born infants. The rate of low birth weight increased to 2 percent for infants of white mothers and to 9 percent for infants of black mothers. The poverty rate for children under age 18 continued to increase to 21 percent in 1992. For black children it was 3 times that for white children and for Hispanic children it was 2.4 times that for white children. The pregnancy rates for teenagers appear to have leveled off, with only slight increases in certain urban areas.

368. The answer is B. *(U.S. Public Health Service, pp 1–3.)* The greatest decrease in mortality was for stroke. It is still the third leading cause of death, but it has declined 34 percent during the past decade. This continues the downward trend begun in the 1970s. The rates for black persons over 45 years of age is twice that for white persons. Heart disease, still the leading cause of death, declined 27 percent in the past decade, also continuing the downward trend of the 1970s. Asian persons have a 50 percent lower rate of mortality from heart disease than white persons, and black persons mortality is 42 percent higher. Mortality for unintentional injuries declined 27 percent over the decade and dropped from the fourth to the fifth leading cause of death, the first change in rank in over a decade. The mortality for motor vehicle crashes declined 14 percent. For breast cancer, mortality has remained stable over the past decade at 22.7 per 100,000 population for white women, but increased 20 percent for black women at 27.6 per 100,000 population.

369. The answer is C. *(Sierles, pp 349–351.)* Suicide is the eighth leading cause of death in the general population. Next to lung cancer, it is the second most preventable. Several factors support this claim. The majority of suicidal patients have behavioral or psychiatric disorders that can be treated effectively, and 67 percent of persons who kill themselves have consulted their physician in the month before the suicide (40 percent the prior week). Fifty-four percent have been treated for a psychiatric illness in the year before the suicide, and 31 percent in the final month. This means that physicians, if properly trained, could identify the self-destructive behaviors and the high-risk factors and intervene preventively. It also speaks to the pressing need for more mental health support in the United States.

370. The answer is A. *(Last, 13/e, pp 1114–1116.)* Poverty, the most important social variable in infant mortality, is linked to an almost 50 percent greater risk of both neonatal and postnatal death. Other social variables — such as the educational level, occupation, or income of either the mother or father, or whether the parents are married — can influence the risk of infant mortality, but none is as powerful as poverty. Poverty is also a major contributor to adult morbidity and mortality.

371. The answer is A. *(Hamburg, pp 134–136.)* More than 1 million adolescents become pregnant each year, and mortality related to childbirth is one of the five leading causes of death for this age group. While it is suspected that physiologic immaturity accounts for some of the increased risk, this has not been demonstrated. There is a clear increase in the rate of toxemia (of unknown cause) and also an increased incidence of infections of amniotic fluid, placental abruptions, and prolonged or precipitous labor. Pregnant adolescent mothers endanger not only their own health in delivery and in their future, but also the intrauteral and future health of their child.

372. The answer is D. *(Isselbacher, 13/e, pp 450–451.)* The calories required for physical activity above the needs of basal metabolism depend on the type of activity, the duration of activity, and the size of the person performing it. Some tables show energy expenditures based on the type of activity irrespective of the size of the individual, but allowing for body weight and intensity of the activity is more accurate. In spite of these limitations, tables of energy costs can be useful tools in nutrition and medicine. The energy cost of walking 3 miles per hour is only 2 kcal/kg of body weight above maintenance requirements. Thus, a 60-kg (132-lb) person will burn up 120 calories and a 75-kg (165-lb) person will expend 150 calories. An hour of moderate bicycling will expend about 3.5 kcal/kg (210 calories for the 60-kg person or 260 calories for the 75-kg person). Moderately heavy activity, such as swimming (2 mph), expends 7.0 kcal/kg/h or 420 calories per hour for the 60-kg person and 525 calories for the 75-kg person. Light running will consume 7.5 kcal/kg/h (450 or 562 calories, respectively). Thus, an increase in activity can be another behavioral mechanism for generating a negative energy balance for patients attempting to lose weight.

373. The answer is B. *(Last, 13/e, pp 741–760.)* Alcohol abuse is the second most frequent form of drug dependence after tobacco. It directly affects an estimated 2.5 to 5 percent of the United States population. In addition, their families, employers, and coworkers are directly and indirectly affected. With about half the annual traffic deaths being related to alcohol use and abuse, a major physical health and disability problem is generated. The economic loss associated with alcohol abuse was estimated to be over $100 billion annually (tobacco estimated at $60 billion). Drinking alcoholic beverages has generally become a socially acceptable form of activity, but its adverse effect on health and behavior can be severe. Alcohol use contributes to a number of disease conditions and reduces the efficiency of productive activity. The highest mortality of alcohol abusers is from cirrhosis of the liver, followed by suicide, accidents, and cancer of the upper digestive and respiratory tracts. The average life span of an alcoholic is shortened by 10 to 12 years. The increased use of psychoactive and addictive drugs, especially among the younger age group, has led to a major effort to bring such drug dependence into the mainstream of modern medicine, public health, and medical education. Furthermore, there is a renewed recognition of both the physical and psychological dependence common with the use of alcohol and tobacco. Although alcohol-related problems of the heavy drinker are more frequent, the moderately drinking segment of the population is actually a much larger group and contributes the greater proportion of the problems. Therefore, physicians must be aware of the greater dimension of the problem rather than just focusing on the minority who use alcohol in large quantities.

374. The answer is D. *(Kapstein, pp 132–139.)* After myocardial infarction a patient experiences many psychosocial and physical responses, even a full year after the acute attack. The most frequent response is a change in mood, leading to depression and anxiety. Also, a majority report experiencing moderate physical distress, extensive disturbances in subjective states, contradictions between patients and their families in assessing the patient's level of activity, the perception of themselves as handicapped, and personal lives that have not returned to normal. These factors must be recognized in order to achieve a successful rehabilitation.

375. The answer is D. *(Isselbacher, 13/e, pp 27–28.)* Suicide is relatively uncommon before puberty. It is the fourth leading cause of death from ages 10 to 14 and becomes the second leading cause of death (after motor vehicle accidents) from the ages of 18 to 24. The highest rates of suicide are found in white and Native American males. It is important to recognize that for every suicide there are between 50 and 120 attempted suicides; attempts are more frequent among females. Drug ingestion is the most common method for attempted suicide in adolescents, but it is usually not fatal. Fatal suicide usually involves firearms, hanging, or jumping from heights. The most common behavioral and psychosocial factors include a family history of suicide, alcohol and substance abuse, conduct disorders, depression, anxiety states, and knowing someone who has attempted or committed suicide. Precipitating factors include acute stress, trouble with the law, trouble at school (e.g., cheating or truancy), substance abuse, pregnancy or fear of pregnancy, hypochondriasis, social isolation, and anxiety. Physicians should recognize that the most important underlying psychological factor in suicidal adolescents is depression, with feelings of hopelessness, low self-esteem, despair, and somatic complaints.

376. The answer is E. *(Isselbacher, 13/e, pp 14–18.)* Ischemic heart disease (IHD) is the leading cause of death among women (nearly 400,000 deaths annually). The death rate is 5 to 6 times that for lung or breast cancer. Because men develop IHD 10 years earlier than women and die of IHD 20 years earlier, many persons think of IHD as primarily a problem of men. High-density lipoprotein (HDL) cholesterol levels are about 10 mg/dL higher in women in all age groups, and there is some evidence that HDL may be more related to IHD among women than low-density lipoprotein (LDL). The relative power of various risk factors and the extent to which interventions prescribed for men can change a woman's risk need more study. Obesity, smoking, hypertension, and oral contraceptives are risk factors for IHD in women.

377. The answer is E. *(Sierles, pp 163–164.)* The fastest growing age group in the United States is the group 80 years old and older. This is attributed to increased health concerns and better medical care. The number of persons over 65 years of age now exceeds the number of persons aged 25 years or younger. A significant problem for medicine is that this group requires more medical care and greater costs primarily for chronic illnesses. Women outlive men by a ratio of 1.5:1 and they also have a greater utilization of health care than men.

378. The answer is C. *(Isselbacher, 13/e, pp 7–8.)* On a general hospital service, only about 15 percent of patients given cardiopulmonary resuscitation (CPR) survive to discharge. Hospital patients are increasingly concerned that they will be subjected to abusive modern technology. While CPR has a definite role in some emergency situations, in a hospital setting it should be discussed in advance. In general, it will be attempted unless a "do not resuscitate" (DNR) order has been made. DNR orders are appropriate if requested, especially if CPR would most likely be futile. "Slow" or "show" codes that merely appear to provide CPR are deceptive and should be questioned on an ethical basis. Sometimes patients may need to be reassured that DNR signifies that only CPR will be withheld and does not mean that other appropriate care or procedures will be withheld.

379. The answer is C. *(Sierles, pp 277–286.)* Dementia is a "falling away of the mind." The prevalence of severe dementia is 1.0 to 1.3 percent, and 15 percent of persons aged 65 years or older suffer from dementia. The most common cause of dementia is Alzheimer's disease, which constitutes 50 to 60 percent of all dementias. Onset is very slow, and prevalence increases with age (5 percent at age 65 to 20 to 50 percent at age 90). It is familial and progresses from stage 1, where speech and memory are affected and a depressive mood is common. In stage 2 there is progression of cognitive and memory deterioration and sensory aphasia; patients often lose their way, and constructional abilities and other praxic functions decline. In stage 3 sphincter control is lost, limbs become rigid and flexed, speech is lost or limited to verbigeration or echolalia, and death usually ensues from aspiration pneumonia or urinary tract infection. Multiple small cerebral infarctions are the second most common cause of dementia (10 percent) and are related to arteriosclerosis, hypertension, diabetes mellitus, and smoking. Multi-infarct dementia has a relatively sudden onset. The gradual degeneration from Pick's disease (cause unknown) accounts for 5 percent of the dementias. Next in frequency are dementias associated with disease of the basal ganglia (Huntington's, Parkinson's and Wilson's), hydrocephalic dementias (with an excess of spinal fluid in the cranial cavity), and dementias associated with infections (e.g., viral dementias of AIDS and bacterial dementias like that of syphilis). Psychiatric dementias sometimes occur in elderly patients who have a major depression with melancholia and with psychomotor slowing and bowed posture, but these can be reversed by cyclic antidepressants or electroconvulsive therapy.

380. The answer is D. *(Hazzard, 3/e, pp 153–164.)* Heart disease is the leading cause of death both in the general and the elderly population. Cancer ranks second and cerebrovascular disease ranks third among the elderly. The fourth leading cause of death for persons age 65 and over is chronic obstructive pulmonary disease, followed by pneumonia, diabetes, and accidents. Suicide is an important cause of mortality, especially among elderly depressed males, but it is not among the 10 leading causes of death of persons age 65 and over.

381. The answer is C. *(Rosen, pp 72–73.)* Obesity increases risks for both physical and psychological disorders. It has been well documented as a primary contributing factor in the development of adult-onset diabetes, hypertension, myocardial hypertrophy, arthritis, gout, menstrual abnormalities, and reproductive problems. It is also a secondary contributing factor in endometrial cancer. It is related to gallbladder disease, but primarily on a correlational basis.

382. The answer is D. *(Isselbacher, 13/e, pp 446–452.)* Fat will accumulate only when the intake of energy exceeds the output of energy. The major causes of obesity have been found to be social, environmental, psychological, economic, ethnic, cultural, racial, genetic, metabolic, endocrinologic, and nutritional. Although studies have not identified any consistent personality factor common to obese persons, the psychological makeup of obese persons has a definite influence on their difficulty in making a satisfactory weight or diet adjustment. Some behavioral factors include life-style, life adjustment, emotional support, anxiety relief, substitute for love and security, response to or defense against tension and frustration, availability of food, comfortable environment, linking of food and hospitality, eating habits, decreased activity, and conditions under which one usually eats. Analysis of these factors and programs to change these behaviors have been found to facilitate weight control.

383. The answer is B. *(Hazzard, 3/e, pp 135–150, 187–190.)* Medical technology and modern medicine (primarily pharmaceutical) have clearly contributed to the decline of certain diseases, but changes in life-style and, in some instances, environment have had the greatest impact on the major diseases over time. Infectious diseases were already declining decades before the discovery of antibiotics. Tuberculosis declined throughout the century before specific antimicrobial agents were introduced. Rheumatic heart disease was also declining because of better living conditions before penicillin was discovered. The decline of coronary artery disease was effected by life-style changes before acute coronary care and intensive care units, coronary artery bypass surgery, and angioplasty were developed. Likewise, cerebrovascular disease, or stroke, has been declining since about 1915. The life-style changes that have had the most effect on these and many other diseases are those involving diet (e.g., consumption of fats and salt), smoking, exercise, stress, environmental toxins, and the prevention and reduction of hypertension. While carcinoma of the prostate is the third most common cause of cancer mortality in men, its etiology is unknown and treatment seems to have little effect on mortality. To date, it has not been associated with life-style, although environmental factors have been implicated.

384. The answer is D. *(Schneiderman, pp 243–249.)* Behavioral methods have been developed to treat both the psychological and physiologic aspects of many diseases that have been formerly regarded as exclusively organic. Of the treatments for cardiovascular diseases, those for hypertension and arrhythmias have successfully benefited from behavioral interventions. In hypertension (particularly mild hypertension), relaxation procedures have been effective in controlling pressure and producing a decrease of 5 to 12 mmHg. Arrhythmias can be regulated by biofeedback and relaxation in some patients, and heart rate can be controlled in most patients. Heart block cannot be controlled, particularly third-degree heart block, in which neural control of heart rate is not possible. However, behavioral intervention can be a judicious adjunct to drugs and other treatments. Raynaud's disease (and migraine headache) can be effectively treated with temperature biofeedback and relaxation procedures. Asthma has been treated in some patients by relaxation, self-control, and stress control. Placebo effects are also helpful. Asthma and hypertension, as well as many other diseases, can be treated effectively with behavioral intervention and conjoint use of drugs and other treatments.

385. The answer is B. *(Kandel, 3/e, pp 1001–1002.)* Food aversion (also called *bait shyness* in animals) is a basic biologic process in which persons learn to avoid poisoned substances. The person develops an aversion to food that is followed by nausea produced by a poison. The food aversion paradigm has been applied to the treatment of chronic alcoholism when alcohol is followed by a powerful emetic such as apomorphine. The same mechanism appears to be involved when a person with Addison's disease becomes conditioned to avoid diets deficient in salt and diets that produce malaise. Certain forms of cancer also produce malaise that induces food aversion and depressed appetite. The nausea following chemotherapy for cancer also produces an aversion to foods tasted before the treatment. Anticipatory nausea can also occur before chemotherapy through conditioning mechanisms, so that the sight of the clinic, smell of the clinic, or even anticipating the visit can induce nausea.

386. The answer is C. *(Rosen, p 8.)* The social and economic characteristics of a population, such as income, education, and marital status, are better predictors of morbidity and longevity than biologic or psychological markers. Sex and age, however, are the exceptions. Over the life span, the frequency of disease and mortality increases. Also, women retain an advantage of approximately 8 years over men in longevity.

387. The answer is D. *(Williams, RB, pp 90–94.)* Behavioral factors influence the development of coronary heart disease through the cardiovascular or endocrine correlates of sympathetic-adrenal-medullary and pituitary-adrenal-cortical activity. The following mechanisms are currently considered to be most involved: (1) behavioral stressors can promote arterial injury through hemodynamic forces, such as turbulence and sheer stress caused by repeated physiologic reactions of excessive heart rate and pressor response; (2) biochemical sources of injury may exert toxic influences on coronary arteries through behaviorally caused increases in endocrines such as catecholamines and corticosteroids; (3) increased circulating catecholamines may affect atherogenesis through influences on platelet aggregation and on the mobilization of serum lipids; (4) acute behavioral stressors can lower the thresholds for ventricular fibrillation; and (5) central nervous system control of the heart can initiate arrhythmic activity, potentially precipitating sudden cardiac death.

388. The answer is B. *(Rosen, pp 18–29.)* Twelve percent of teenagers 12 to 17 years old smoke, which increases to 26 percent for those 17 to 18 years old. About one-third of all 18 year olds are regular smokers. While the teenage smoking rates appear to be decreasing, it may be that only the older group has leveled off. It is important to recognize that the age for beginning smoking is decreasing, especially for females. Sixty percent of the female smokers begin smoking before they are 13 years of age.

389. The answer is D. *(Rosen, pp 119–120.)* Studies of males involved in aerobic-type exercise and jogging have reported a significant reduction in anxiety, depression, and hostility when these males are compared with sedentary controls. They have also reported greater self-confidence. Type A males also showed a reduction in type A patterns of behavior. Biologic stress-reducing factors that could influence such psychological factors are the usual reduction of circulating catecholamines and the increase in β-endorphins occurring during exercise.

390. The answer is D. *(Hazzard, 3/e, pp 167–175.)* Treatment with multiple medications is a major health problem in the elderly and enhances the hazard of complications from those drugs. About 90 percent of the elderly take at least one medication and the majority take two or more. Forty percent are over-the-counter drugs. It has also been found that over half of patients over age 60 make one or more medication errors during each illness. Psychotropic agents surpass all other drugs consumed in long-term care facilities (in 75 percent of institutionalized patients as opposed to 35 percent of ambulatory patients). The highest risk factors for adverse drug reactions, in addition to use of multiple drugs, include being a woman; this risk is most frequently attributed to small body size. Although only 12 percent of the American population is over age 65, this group consumes 20 to 25 percent of the total national drug expenditure. This is expected to increase in the future.

391. The answer is B. *(Gatchel, 2/e, pp 69–72.)* The stress of various life events or changes is known to correlate highly with the development of various illnesses. Not all life events are of equal importance, but three general characteristics of important life events have been identified; desirability of an event, control, and required adjustment. If an event is highly undesirable, it is more stressful. If a person feels very little or no control over the event, it is more stressful. Likewise, an event is more stressful if a great amount of effort is required to cope with it. The frequency of a threatening or stressful event can be linked to an illness, not necessarily through the severity of the threat, but through its chronic or "hassle" effect. Reappraisal is an ongoing process, but not a general characteristic linking the stress of life events to illness.

392. The answer is A. *(Kandel, 3/e, pp 805–810.)* The inability to sleep is a hardship that can alter a person's mood and behavior and even disrupt a life by affecting the entire behavioral repertoire. Quantitative surveys have established that about one in five persons has a sleep problem. Physicians report that the two most common complaints in medicine are pain and trouble sleeping. Insomnia is defined as the chronic inability to obtain the necessary amount or quality of sleep to maintain adequate daytime behavior. In reality it is a symptom of a variety of disorders. It is such a public health problem that there is an excessive tendency of poor sleepers to medicate themselves and for physicians to overprescribe strong sleeping pills. The net result is a serious problem of abuse of sleeping medications. Various studies have shown that there is very little evidence that any current sleeping medication is effective for more than several days. A part of the reason for so much overtreatment of sleep complaints is that they are often exaggerated by patients.

393. The answer is C. *(Gatchel, 2/e, pp 39–49.)* During World War II, researchers noticed that Londoners showed increased blood pressure during the early phases of the mass bombings. Also, studies of incarceration in German concentration camps and prisoner-of-war camps found that survivors showed greater rates of physical illness and greater rates of relatively permanent problems of psychological adjustment than people of similar age who were not prisoners. The incidence of premature death was also higher in survivors of concentration camps during the years following their release. One study found that survivors of concentration camps who had developed cancer were poorer at coping than similar patients who had not been in camps. Thus, such survivors may have been more vulnerable to stress associated with cancer.

394. The answer is B. *(Isselbacher, 13/e, pp 2420–2421.)* It is estimated that 90 percent of people in the U.S. drink alcohol at some time, 40 to 50 percent of men have temporary alcohol-induced problems, and 10 percent of men and 3 to 5 percent of women develop alcoholism. Even light drinking can adversely interact with other medications, heavier drinking can exacerbate most medical illnesses, and alcoholism can masquerade as other medical disorders and psychiatric syndromes. While most information on alcohol applies to the "average" person, there is considerable variability among individuals that depends on genetic factors, other drug use, and existing pathology or disease. It is also little appreciated that the cancer rate with alcoholism is 10 times higher than that in the general population, especially in the head and neck, esophagus, stomach, liver, and pancreas. The homeless or skid-row alcoholic represents only 5 percent or less of all alcoholics. In general, 12 oz of beer, 4 oz of non-fortified wine, and 1.5 oz of 80-proof beverage contain the same amount (10 g) of ethanol.

395. The answer is E. *(Hamburg, p 133.)* Anorexia nervosa is an emotional disorder of adolescent females that is life-threatening. There is self-imposed starvation that may require hospitalization. The pathogenesis of anorexia is still not completely understood, but it does involve family relations, a disturbed body image, need for overachievement, and a concern for control and sexuality; it also often involves depression. The very difficult treatment of anorexia often involves a combination of modalities, such as hospitalization, medically regulated feeding, behavior modification, antidepressant drugs, and psychotherapy. Anorexia nervosa is a very complex, life-threatening disorder and is not simply a case of dieting out of control.

396. The answer is B. *(Rosen, pp 303–304.)* Although a "cancer-prone personality" has not been identified, the link between behavior and cancer progression is becoming more established, especially for the relationship between the inability to express emotion (e.g., hostility) and cancer. Sandra Levy is finding that negatively reactive patients with metastatic breast cancer live significantly longer than passive patients. Negative reactivity does not imply obnoxious behavior but rather a determination to "fight" the cancer and begin to cope positively versus giving way to apathy, helplessness, or surrender. On the other hand, overly cooperative, bland, and passive cancer patients in the face of stress have a shorter life span. Also, patients with breast cancer who are married or who are a part of an intact social network have an increased survival rate. Depression will act to suppress the immune system and thus will not assist longer survival.

397. The answer is E. *(Last, 13/e, pp 688–694.)* Symptoms of physical illness that might be defined simply as perceived or subjective changes of one's bodily state play a key role in health care. Such perceived changes, combined with observable signs, are the only way that the presence of illness can be detected. An understanding of how these symptoms and signs are interpreted by the average person is important for the practicing physician. The traditional view concerning the frequency of symptoms states that the illness experience constitutes a relatively infrequent or unusual event. In recent years, however, there have been a number of studies of symptom prevalence in normal populations; this evidence shows that there is a sizable number of clinically serious problems reported in supposedly healthy populations. Various empirical studies have reported that a wide range of symptoms—including headaches, upset stomachs, sore muscles, chest pains, nasal congestion, watering eyes, ringing in the ears, racing heart, dizziness, flushed face, sweating hands, and shortness of breath—occurs frequently and that many if not most people experience some of these symptoms much of the time. Behavioral scientists have also found that only a small number of people experiencing such problems ever seek professional care. In most cases, the mere presence of symptoms does not prompt a person to seek professional assistance. Illness becomes an everyday typical experience, and the treated case actually represents only the tip of a clinical iceberg. It is further evident that the experience of unexpected physiologic arousal (symptoms) places a person in a position of needing and seeking information from others to help give meaning to what he or she is experiencing. Thus, when unexpected physiologic changes occur, research findings suggest that we seek out explanations or attributions from our memory and through the advice of others.

398. The answer is E. *(Gatchel, 2/e, p 238.)* A placebo effect is any nonspecific, psychologic, or psychophysiologic therapeutic effect produced by a supposedly inert substance or nontherapeutic treatment. It is most often based on the belief or expectations of patients that the placebo will help them or relieve their symptoms. Historically, the placebo played a major role in medical treatment before the discovery of modern pharmacologic agents. The placebo effect is useful in psychotherapy, especially in the treatment of anxiety, and has also been shown to be an important factor in the biofeedback process. Endorphins (endogenous opiate-like substances in the brain) are involved in the mediation of the placebo effect. There is extensive literature in the research journals verifying the fact that the belief of the patient that a prescribed medication is active (even if it is chemically inert) often leads to significant reduction of symptoms, including a reduction in pain. The placebo also plays a role when used with modern chemically active and inactive drugs.

399. The answer is D. *(Kaplan, 7/e, pp 371, 762, 772.)* Hyperthyroidism (thyrotoxicosis) is a syndrome resulting from a chronic excess of thyroid hormone (thyroxine). It may be precipitated by acute emotional stress and may even develop within hours after an emotional trauma. It is an endocrine disorder and is almost always accompanied by mental changes—the patient may feel tense and hyperexcitable and may be emotionally labile, with inappropriate temper outbursts, crying spells, or euphoria. Distractibility, short attention span, and impaired recent memory may also be present. Severe hyperthyroidism may result in frank psychosis, delirium, coma, and death. Thyroid disorders are seven times more frequent in women than in men; they occur most commonly in women in their third and fourth decades and in men at older ages. In contrast to the tense and hyperexcitable behaviors usually observed, a minority of patients, particularly the elderly, may be depressed, apathetic, and anorectic with chronic hyperthyroidism. Mildly hyperthyroid patients occasionally are misdiagnosed as having anxiety neuroses. Mental retardation in children is frequently associated with hypothyroidism, not hyperthyroidism, since normal brain development requires the thyroid hormone.

400. The answer is B. *(Rosen, pp 132–133.)* In the type A pattern of behavior, the joyless striving characteristic is regarded by Friedman and Rosenman as representing a constant struggle for recognition and reward in order to overcome fears of inadequacy and insecurity. As such, emotional exhaustion, feelings of despair, hopelessness, and depression can be recognized as prodromes in type A persons just prior to their myocardial infarction and frequently sudden death. Such chronic striving can represent an attempt to overcome the underlying feelings of depression. Disregarding time pressures would actually be therapeutic, especially for a person with a strong type A personality.

401. The answer is D. *(Isselbacher, 13/e, pp 23–30.)* Even though adolescents are relatively free of illnesses and have lower rates of illness and use of health care than children or adults, they account for over twice as many automobile accidents as adults, 20 percent of all suicides, well over 600,000 pregnancies in unmarried girls per year, and a 32 percent pregnancy rate among sexually active, unmarried teenagers. They are the only age group for which the death rate is actually increasing, with a higher death rate than 20 years ago. Seventy percent of all deaths of teenagers are the result of automobile accidents or violence, both of which are increasing in frequency among adolescents while they are decreasing in the general population. The reported smoking rate for persons 12 to 17 years old is 12 percent; the rate increases to 26 percent for those 17 to 18 years old.

402. The answer is D. *(Last, 13/e, pp 671–723.)* The health consequences of smoking behavior are well established and clearly understood. The term *smoking behavior* is used because smoking is a behavioral act. Studies show that smokers, especially cigarette smokers, are much more likely than nonsmokers to die from a large number of diseases. Among these are diseases of the heart, bronchitis/emphysema, arteriosclerosis, and cancers of the lung, oral cavity, larynx, pancreas, bladder, esophagus, and kidney. Other diseases and disorders caused or affected by smoking behavior are cancer of the upper gastrointestinal tract, peptic ulcers, and adverse effects on the fetus. Increases in total mortality of cigarette smokers in prospective studies vary from 30 to 80 percent, depending partly on the age groups studied. An overall risk of 60 per-

cent greater than the mortality of nonsmokers is considered a reasonable estimate. This results in a reduced life expectancy of cigarette smokers of 5 to 6
years. The reduction in life expectancy increases directly with the number of
cigarettes smoked. Between 1970 and 1985, deaths from lung cancer among
women 55 to 74 years of age increased about 7 percent each year compared
with a 1 percent increase for men. Since 1987, mortality from lung cancer
among women has exceeded that from breast cancer. While there has been a
reduction in the number of male smokers, the number of female smokers is
still increasing. Lung cancer deaths attributed to smoking addiction appear to
have peaked for males. The death rate for females is still climbing rapidly.

403. The answer is D. *(Gatchel, 2/e, pp 56–58.)* Most studies dealing with
the effects of exercise on depression have demonstrated significant improvements in the subject's mood state. Exercise was as effective as time-limited
psychotherapy, mediation, or group psychotherapy. Exercise fostered a sense
of mastery, a positive self-image, an increased peripheral and cerebral blood
flow, increased oxygenation, increased levels of catecholamines (norepinephrine and epinephrine), and some cathartic relief. While the studies have been
mainly correlational rather than causative and they may have been influenced
by a self-selecting bias, the evidence is considered more than suggestive. The
expectancy and demand characteristics associated with exercise are very powerful.

404. The answer is E. *(U.S. Public Health Service, pp 1, 12, 69, 73.)* Survival is not the sole criterion for evaluating outcomes of pregnancy. Many
conditions that may lead to an infant's death also carry potential hazardous
consequences when the outcome is not fatal. The most significant characteristic associated with a poor outcome of pregnancy is low birth weight, usually
defined as less than $5 \frac{1}{2}$ pounds (2500 g). Infants of low birth weight face a
fiftyfold greater chance of dying before 1 month of age and are five times
more likely to die between 1 month and 1 year of age than are infants of normal birth weight. They are also more likely to have serious congenital anomalies or other severe impairments. Babies of low birth weight are likely to
have a greater rate of developmental problems than are heavier babies. The
morbidity and mortality of low birth weight are most frequently related to
poverty, lack of prenatal care, poor nutrition, smoking, stress, and poor physical condition. In 1991, 7.1 percent of all infants born in the United States were
of low birth weight. The incidence of low birth weight was more than twice as
high for black infants as it was for white infants (13.6 percent and 5.8 percent,
respectively). Nearly all the difference in neonatal mortality between white
and black infants can be attributed to difference in the distribution of birth
weight. The regions that achieved lower rates than the U.S. average for infants

of low birth weight were the Pacific, New England, West North Central, and Mountain regions with 5.81, 5.97, 5.97, and 6.76 per 100 live births, respectively. The others ranged between 7.39 and 8.30 per 100 live births.

405. The answer is D. *(Kaplan, 7/e, pp 1120–1122, 1153–1154.)* During adolescence, there is a marked increase in the number of suicides. Adolescents account for 6000 of the 28,000 yearly suicides in the United States. Boys are three times more likely to commit suicide than are girls, and boys typically choose more violent acts than the more passive methods used by girls. Suicide is the third leading cause of death among adolescents, exceeded only by accidents and homicides. It is thought that suicide attempts represent an adolescent's final call for help and attention. These attempts are all too often successful. During the period between 1970 and 1980, the rate of suicide for adolescent males increased 40 percent and is still rising. The suicide rate for females is also continuing to rise. Studies show that 60 percent of adolescents who commit suicide live with only one parent. Suicide risk is also associated with depression, with families in which one or more members has a chronic illness, with a family history of suicide, and with long-standing family and social problems throughout childhood. Suicide can be precipitated by another suicide in a peer group, by a loss of a loved one, and by an adolescent suicide seen on television. A substrate of psychopathology generally exists.

406. The answer is C. *(Isselbacher, 13/e, pp 2420–2425.)* The diagnosis of alcoholism is difficult. General criteria include four situations: when a person ignores early warning signs such as alcohol-related problems in marriage and then goes on to an alcohol-related marital separation or divorce; when a person is fired or laid off because of an alcohol-related problem; when there are two or more arrests related to alcohol; or when there is evidence that alcohol has harmed one's health, such as cardiomyopathy, cirrhosis, or alcoholic hepatitis, including signs of alcohol withdrawal. If a person has alcohol-related problems during an episode of mania or related to a preexisting antisocial personality disorder, then the alcohol problem is likely to be secondary to the primary disorder and not alcoholism per se.

407–410. The answers are 407-E, 408-C, 409-B, 410-A. *(Isselbacher, 13/e, pp 199–203, 1735–1738, 2119–2122, 1692–1698.)* Sickle cell anemia is a congenital hemolytic anemia seen most frequently among, and hence characterized as a condition of, the black population. About 0.15 percent of black children in the United States have sickle cell anemia. It has a lower prevalence in adults because of decreased life expectancy.

Phenylketonuria is an autosomal recessive metabolic disorder. It is associated with severe mental retardation and, less frequently, with other neurologic manifestations such as psychomotor symptoms. No abnormalities are apparent at birth, but treatment in early infancy may prevent retardation.

Osteoarthritis, known also as *degenerative joint disease*, is most often an affliction of advancing years. Wear-and-tear processes seem to be the major causative factor; certain occupations and hobbies, particularly those involving joint trauma, appear to be causally related to the development of osteoarthritis. Forty million Americans have radiologic evidence of degenerative joint disease, including 85 percent of persons over the age of 70.

Although dental decay has links with heredity and a direct relationship to age, the most important factor associated with tooth decay at every age is lack of attention and poor oral hygiene, most frequently occurring in poverty or lower socioeconomic situations. Unless treated, this infection of enamel and underlying dentin in due course extends to involvement of the dental pulp and frequently results in loss of the affected tooth.

Behavioral Risk Factors and Disease

DIRECTIONS: Each question below contains five suggested responses. Select the **one best** response to each question.

411. The single most significant source of preventable morbidity and premature mortality is

(A) environmental pollution
(B) crime and homicide
(C) auto and home accidents
(D) poor nutrition
(E) cigarette smoking

412. The most effective behavioral intervention for hypertension is

(A) biofeedback
(B) relaxation
(C) learning to discriminate sources of stress
(D) developing alternative reactions to stressors
(E) diet

413. The principle of covariation of risk behaviors means that

(A) risk behaviors usually occur together or at the same time
(B) a high-risk behavior can become extinct by reviving and reinforcing a former behavior of lower risk
(C) the onset of one risk behavior is associated with the subsequent initiation of another
(D) there is a relatively equal potential that either of two risk behaviors will occur at any one time
(E) the practice (expression) of one risk behavior triggers another risk behavior

414. It has been found that there is a higher incidence of stress-related coronary heart disease among

(A) women working outside the home in general than among housewives
(B) childless women working outside the home than among housewives in general
(C) working women with control over decisions than working women with little input on decisions
(D) clerical workers than among housewives
(E) housewives with several children than among women working outside the home with fewer children

415. In the next decade, the best hope for controlling the HIV epidemic is through

(A) reducing the incidence and prevalence of intravenous drug use
(B) changing sexual behaviors
(C) increasing adherence to HIV/AIDS treatment regimens
(D) educating the public about HIV/AIDS
(E) promoting the development and testing of an effective drug to cure AIDS

416. True statements related to AIDS and ARC (AIDS-related complex) include

(A) the minority of intravenous drug users share needles regularly
(B) the time needed for reported cases to double has increased modestly with increased public education
(C) the manner in which AIDS is transmitted can be characterized as primarily behavioral
(D) the spreading of AIDS into the heterosexual community has recently begun to level off
(E) the only existing palliative treatment is AZT

417. The component of the type A pattern of behavior most pathogenic for coronary heart disease is

(A) physiologic reactivity to social stress
(B) impatience
(C) vigorous speech
(D) hostility
(E) competitive drive

418. Which of the following actions would most powerfully reduce the incidence of cardiovascular disease?

(A) Reduction of salt intake
(B) Reduction of excess weight
(C) Exercise
(D) Reduction of type A behavior
(E) Cessation of cigarette smoking

419. The risk behavior most often associated with motor vehicle accidents and injuries during adolescence is

(A) use of illicit drugs
(B) use of alcohol
(C) reckless driving
(D) failure to use seat belts
(E) failure to use helmets

420. What percentage of the mortality from the 10 leading causes of death in the United States can be traced to life-style?

(A) 10
(B) 20
(C) 30
(D) 40
(E) 50

421. The leading cause of death for African-American male adolescents is

(A) motor vehicle accidents
(B) homicide
(C) suicide
(D) genetic and developmental cardiovascular disease
(E) alcohol and substance abuse

422. Most of the major health problems of adolescents

(A) have a genetic basis
(B) have a sexual basis
(C) involve sensory deficits
(D) are self-inflicted
(E) involve bacterial and viral infections

423. The best predictor of health and longevity is

(A) income level
(B) education level
(C) life-style
(D) marital status
(E) religious participation

424. In comparing the rates of motor vehicle accidents of patients who have been hospitalized for mental illness with those of patients who have chronic systemic illnesses, the mentally ill group had

(A) three times as many
(B) twice as many
(C) 50 percent more
(D) the same number
(E) 50 percent less

425. A gun kept at home for protection is most likely to be involved in

(A) the death of the homeowner
(B) the killing of an intruder
(C) an accidental death
(D) the killing of a family member
(E) a suicide

426. The major cause of death among adolescents and young adults is

(A) homicide
(B) suicide
(C) motor vehicle accidents
(D) infections
(E) illicit drug abuse

427. Which of the following statements about smoking is true?

(A) The most effective deterrent to substance abuse is arousal of fear

(B) The major influence on teenagers to smoke comes from their parents

(C) The social context is the excuse, not the reason, for maintaining a smoking habit

(D) The most rapid increase in smoking is among teenage females

(E) Social inoculation strategy in prevention has not been effective

428. Stress leading to the risk of psychosomatic disorders can be best measured by the

(A) Friedman and Rosenman structured interview

(B) Luria-Nebraska battery

(C) Minnesota multiphasic personality inventory

(D) Holmes and Rahe rating scale

(E) Rorschach test

DIRECTIONS: Each numbered question or incomplete statement below is NEGATIVELY phrased. Select the **one best** lettered response.

429. Human immunodeficiency virus (HIV) is spread primarily by all the following EXCEPT

(A) exchange of bodily fluids during sex
(B) sharing of needles or other drug paraphernalia
(C) blood transfusion
(D) fomites contaminated by respiratory infection
(E) perinatal contact of an infected mother with her infant

430. Alcohol consumption in pregnant females is associated with all the following risks for the infant EXCEPT

(A) fetal alcohol syndrome in 1 per 1000 live births
(B) decreased birth weight
(C) mental retardation
(D) increased spontaneous abortion
(E) poor sucking ability

431. True statements regarding adolescence include all the following EXCEPT

(A) mortality is generally higher for males
(B) accidents are positively correlated with affluence
(C) accidents are the leading cause of death among males
(D) at least half of motor vehicle accidents involve alcohol
(E) suicide is the leading cause of death among females

432. All the following social and cultural factors have been found to be related to the development of hypertension EXCEPT

(A) stress
(B) personality
(C) obesity
(D) dietary salt
(E) compliance with medical treatment

433. Duodenal ulcer activity is exacerbated by all the following EXCEPT

(A) expression of a characteristic personality
(B) chronic anxiety
(C) alcohol consumption
(D) psychological stress
(E) cigarette smoking

434. Chronic alcohol consumption by a pregnant woman can produce fetal alcohol syndrome. Which of the following symptoms is LEAST likely?

(A) Retardation of intrauterine growth
(B) Defective cerebral development
(C) Microcephaly
(D) Premature birth
(E) Reduction in number of fingers and toes

435. Risk factors for problem behaviors in adolescence can be identified. All the following personal or personality factors have a major influence EXCEPT

(A) unconventionality
(B) rebelliousness
(C) high risk-taking
(D) low value on achievement
(E) low value on autonomy

436. An adolescent has an increased risk of becoming a smoker if all the following are true EXCEPT that he or she

(A) is employed outside the home
(B) has a high level of achievement in school
(C) has parents who smoke
(D) has friends who smoke
(E) has adult role models who smoke

437. College students are considered to be at risk for AIDS because of all the following EXCEPT

(A) frequent sexual contact
(B) a sense of invulnerability
(C) the belief that only homosexuals and drug users get AIDS
(D) the belief that educated people are not apt to get AIDS
(E) a lack of knowledge about risks

438. Correct statements about insomnia include all the following EXCEPT

(A) the most common causes of insomnia are psychological and emotional disturbances
(B) anxiety is positively correlated with difficulty in falling asleep
(C) depression is positively correlated with frequency of early awakenings
(D) the most frequent emotional cause of insomnia is anxiety
(E) anticipation of poor sleep is the cause in about 15 percent of cases

439. Failure to cope with psychological stress has been found to contribute rather consistently to the pathogenesis of all the following illnesses EXCEPT

(A) coronary artery disease
(B) hypertension
(C) gastrointestinal problems
(D) cancer
(E) alcohol abuse

440. Research findings on the use of alcoholic beverages show all the following EXCEPT

(A) the alcoholic's life span is shortened by 10 to 12 years
(B) alcohol is considered to be a contributory cause in half of all deaths resulting from automobile accidents
(C) total abstinence represents the predominant disease model approach to treatment
(D) the social learning model has not been shown to be effective for treating problem drinking and alcoholism
(E) the usual public policy response to alcohol-related health problems is to increase treatment services

441. Of the following behavioral factors, which is LEAST likely to enhance tumor growth?

(A) Bereavement
(B) Consumption of alcohol
(C) Exercise
(D) Stress
(E) Lack of close personal ties

442. Great potential for health promotion exists in all the following strategies EXCEPT

(A) changing the typical stance of dependence in the relationship with professionals
(B) development of more healthful patterns of daily living
(C) mitigating and eliminating risk factors
(D) more effective adaptation to the presence of chronic illness
(E) increased use of physician services

443. *Life-style* refers to those individual and societal patterns of behavior that are at least partly under individual control and that demonstrably influence personal health. True statements regarding health status and life-style behaviors include all the following EXCEPT

(A) the major causes of death, serious illness, and disability in the United States today are chronic disease and violence

(B) the underlying causes of most chronic disease, disability, and premature death are life-style factors that are potentially amenable to change

(C) a few life-style behaviors (e.g., smoking, drinking alcohol, lack of exercise, and poor eating habits) constitute the major behavioral risk factors involved in chronic disease and severe disability

(D) behavioral techniques that modify life-style patterns can improve both preventive and curative medical practices

(E) changing one's life-style is primarily dependent on an understanding of the risks to one's health and the health behaviors required to reduce those risks

444. True statements about the health consequences of smoking include all the following EXCEPT

(A) the overall mortality risk is 60 percent greater for smokers than for nonsmokers

(B) the risk of dying of lung cancer is between 8 and 15 times higher in a cigarette smoker than in a nonsmoker

(C) life span is shortened by about 5.5 min for each cigarette smoked

(D) children whose parents smoke have a higher incidence of respiratory infections and impaired function than those whose parents do not smoke

(E) while more women than men are initiating smoking, more women are quitting smoking than men

445. All the following statements about obesity are true EXCEPT

(A) obesity increases the risk of developing diabetes approximately fourfold

(B) obese persons are more likely to die in automobile accidents than are members of the population in general

(C) obesity increases the severity of most health problems

(D) obesity is the leading cause of hypertension

(E) obesity has been linked to complications from surgery and infections

446. Exercise has been demonstrated to aid in the prevention of all the following EXCEPT

(A) chronic obstructive lung disease
(B) abnormal body weight and composition
(C) osteoporosis
(D) coronary heart disease
(E) hypertension

447. True statements regarding exercise of moderate intensity include all the following EXCEPT

(A) 30 min of exercise will generally result in an energy expenditure of 300 kcal
(B) the metabolic rate remains elevated for several hours after exercise
(C) exercise helps to retain lean body mass in the elderly
(D) when exercise is combined with calorie restriction, a greater weight loss of muscle tissue is accomplished
(E) increased metabolism from exercise combined with restricted calories increases loss of adipose tissue

448. All the following statements about Down's syndrome are true EXCEPT

(A) most affected persons have 47 chromosomes
(B) the incidence of Down's syndrome is related to maternal age
(C) amniocentesis can detect the presence of Down's syndrome before birth
(D) it accounts for approximately 30 percent of retarded children in the United States
(E) most infants born with Down's syndrome die at an early age

449. All the following are risk factors for cardiovascular disease EXCEPT

(A) physical inactivity
(B) cigarette smoking
(C) obesity
(D) personality type
(E) moderate alcohol consumption

450. Essential hypertension has been frequently associated with all the following EXCEPT

(A) repressed anger
(B) acutely stressful events
(C) familial history of hypertension
(D) decreased sympathetic nervous system activity
(E) decreased parasympathetic inhibition

451. Behavioral factors appear to be crucial to all the following aspects of cigarette smoking EXCEPT

(A) initiation of the smoking habit
(B) maintaining abstinence
(C) day-to-day fluctuations in smoking
(D) nicotine addiction
(E) choice of cigarette brands

452. The importance of psychosocial factors in the etiology of schizophrenia is correctly illustrated by each of the following statements EXCEPT

(A) lower socioeconomic status correlates with a higher incidence of schizophrenia
(B) family psychosocial factors are about equal to biologic factors
(C) the stress-diathesis model has linked biologic vulnerability with induction of stress
(D) there is no schizophrenia-prone personality type
(E) there is a developmental deficit in the vulnerable individual

Behavioral Risk Factors and Disease

Answers

411. The answer is E. *(Last, 13/e, pp 724-726.)* Each U.S. Surgeon General's report since 1964 has emphasized that the single most significant source of preventable morbidity and premature mortality is cigarette smoking. The excess annual toll is estimated to exceed 350,000 people, more than all American lives lost in all wars during the twentieth century. Environmental pollution, crime and homicide, auto and home accidents, and poor nutrition are all significant sources of preventable morbidity and premature death, but smoking is considered the most significant.

412. The answer is B. *(Kaptein, pp 115–123.)* Relaxation training is the most frequently used and the most effective behavioral therapeutic technique for essential hypertension. Of course, relaxation is most effectively used in combination with antihypertensives, but it has demonstrated some lowering of blood pressure, especially in mild hypertensives. Relaxation exercises reduce sympathetic activation and have proved superior to nontreatment, blood pressure self-monitoring, and biofeedback. Learning to discriminate sources of stress, developing alternative reactions to stressors, and diet have all demonstrated some positive effect, but the combination of pharmacotherapy and relaxation training often allows the physician to reduce the medication and also gets the patient involved in the therapeutic process. Relaxation has also been used effectively for prevention.

413. The answer is C. *(Isselbacher, 13/e, p 27.)* The principle of covariation of risk behaviors states that the onset of one risk behavior is associated with, or can be used to predict, the greater likelihood for the initiation of another (usually higher risk) behavior in the future. For example, less serious substance use by an adolescent or young adult can predict the subsequent use of more serious substances. Alcohol use generally precedes use of other illicit drugs. Also, the earlier a person uses alcohol or marijuana, the more likely he or she will move on to more serious drugs. If a person reaches young adulthood without having used these substances, it is unlikely he or she will use them in the future. The major risk for the initiation of cigarette, alcohol, and marijuana use is by age 20 (age 21 for use of other illicit drugs). The initiation of substance use is also correlated with (predictive of) delinquent behavior, early sexual activity, and less effective use of contraceptives. In boys, the initiation of alcohol use is a major predictor of future substance use, sexual activity, and delinquency, while in girls, cigarette use is more predictive of subsequent substance use.

414.   The answer is D. *(Gatchel, 2/e, pp 100–102.)* Occupations with high psychological demands and low control over decisions are associated with increased cardiovascular risk for both men and women. Data from the Framingham Heart Study showed that when working women (employed for more than half of their adult years outside the home) are compared with housewives, in general they were not at significantly higher risk, but clerical workers and working women with children were more apt to develop coronary heart disease. Furthermore, the incidence of coronary heart disease increased linearly with the number of children for working women, but not for housewives with multiple children. Working women whose bosses were nonsupportive were also at greater risk.

415.   The answer is B. *(Sierles, pp 7–13.)* Changing the unprotected sex and other high-risk sexual and social behaviors that promote transmission is the best hope for controlling the HIV epidemic during the next decade. Reducing the incidence and prevalence of intravenous drug use would help control the transmission of the virus through needle sharing, but would still affect only a lesser proportion of the most vulnerable populations. Increasing the adherence to HIV/AIDS treatment regimens would help reduce the morbidity but would not control the transmission, nor is the development and testing of new treatment drugs expected to provide a cure in the next decade. Attempting to educate the public about HIV and AIDS has been modestly successful, but has been grossly inadequate for control of the epidemic.

416.   The answer is C. *(Gatchel, 2/e, pp 138–142.)* The incidence of AIDS has increased rapidly since 1978. It is estimated that three-fourths of AIDS cases occur among gays or bisexuals, followed by intravenous drug users, recipients of transfusion (including hemophiliacs), and children born to mothers infected with HIV. AIDS is increasingly being spread into the heterosexual community, and the time needed for reported cases to double has been decreasing steadily. It has been found that the majority of intravenous drug users share needles regularly. The transmission of AIDS is considered to be potentially controllable using strategies of behavioral change and technologies. There is no cure for AIDS, but powerful drugs and behavioral strategies and technologies can extend life and improve the quality of life.

417. The answer is D. *(Gatchel, 2/e, p 119.)* The type A pattern of behavior has been linked to the risk of coronary heart disease. The specific behavioral factors have been identified as competitiveness, impatience, vigorous speech, hostility, and time urgency. Also, physiologic reactivity to occupational and social stress is a more recently identified component. The hostility component of the type A pattern of behavior has been found to be the most pathogenic of all the behaviors. Hostility, interacting with the other behaviors and stresses, may in effect drive the physiologic reactivity to produce the physiologic and pathologic damage.

418. The answer is E. *(Gatchel, 2/e, pp 97–102.)* There are many physiologic, environmental, and behavioral variables that interact in the development of cardiovascular disease. Age, sex, and family history cannot be controlled, but behavioral and environmental risk factors can be modified by changing a person's life-style. Lowering salt intake, reducing excess weight, increasing exercise, and reducing type A behavior will each assist in lowering the risk, but cessation of smoking has a more powerful effect because it will reduce the severe pathophysiologic effects of smoking.

419. The answer is B. *(Isselbacher, 13/e, pp 26–27.)* More than half of the deaths of adolescents are caused by motor vehicle accidents, and hospitalization for injury consumes the largest number of days spent in the hospital. The use of alcohol plays a significant role in more than half of these accidents and injuries. Next in significance is the high-risk behavior of high-speed and reckless driving. Injuries with bicycles, swimming, skateboards, and boating are also linked to alcohol use and reckless behavior. Failure to use seatbelts and helmets also plays a role in both mortality and morbidity. Illicit drugs are used by 1 to 9 percent of adolescents, but they play a relatively minor role in accidents when compared with the use of alcohol.

420. The answer is E. *(Hamburg, pp 206–207.)* *Life-style* is a term used to refer to single and collective aspects of individual behavior, especially long-term patterns of behavior that characterize a person's general habits of living, adapting, coping, and achieving. The United States Department of Health and Human Services has estimated that 50 percent of the mortality from the 10 leading causes of death can be traced to one's life-style. Major known behavioral risk factors are cigarette smoking, certain dietary habits, reckless driving, violence, use of illicit drugs, excessive consumption of alcoholic beverages, insufficient exercise, nonadherence to medication regimens, maladaptive responses to social pressures and stress, and obesity.

421. The answer is B. *(Isselbacher, 13/e, pp 26–27.)* African-American males 15 to 19 years of age have the lowest life expectancy of all adolescents. They have a fivefold greater rate of death from homicide than white males. Homicide accounts for 40 percent of the deaths in late adolescence and 37 percent in young adults. Living in impoverished metropolitan areas increases the risk tremendously for African-American adolescents. Rates of suicide are lower for African-American than Native American or white adolescents. The rate of death by motor vehicle accident is lower for African-American males than for whites, as is mortality from alcohol and substance abuse. Death from cardiovascular disease is infrequent in adolescents.

422. The answer is D. *(Hamburg, pp 247–256.)* Although most American adolescents judge their own health to be very good, many adolescents take actions that produce self-induced health problems resulting in physical or behavioral disability or death. Most of these have to do with behaviors associated with accidents, drug and alcohol abuse, tobacco use, and poor eating habits. Accidents are the leading cause of death in the adolescent years, and their incidence appears to be increasing at a rapid rate. Homicide is the second leading cause of death, and suicide is the third. Drug, alcohol, and tobacco use usually begin during adolescence or even during preadolescence. Since these activities are all behaviorally related, there is at least the potential that behavioral intervention can make the greatest impact on the health of youth.

423. The answer is C. *(Gatchel, 2/e, pp 290–296.)* A remarkable number of studies have found that life-style, schooling, marital status, income level, and even religious participation are good predictors of health and longevity. While all of these factors are important, life-style represents a combination of all the behavioral factors upon which health risks and prevention are based and has a central role in the etiology and treatment of most diseases. Of course genetics is also a major factor, but one's life-style can have a direct effect on the expression of particular genes or predispositions. Education is associated with income, life changes, life-style, habits, knowledge, self-esteem, and other factors, all of which affect health. Marriage favors men, but both men and women gain significantly relative to unmarried or divorced persons. Religious participation generally is related to conventionality of life-style, and more positive health behaviors in respect to smoking, drinking, and other risks.

424. The answer is D. *(Sierles, p 343.)* The rate of motor vehicle accidents for patients who have been hospitalized for mental illness is about the same as for patients who have chronic systemic illnesses. Alcohol abuse and anti-social and borderline personality disorders were the major factors for the mentally ill group. Personality traits associated with higher frequencies were low tolerance for frustration, emotional instability, aggressiveness, and immaturity. Both the mentally ill group and the chronic systemic illness group still had more motor vehicle accidents than the general population.

425. The answer is E. *(Sierles, pp 359–360.)* Studies show that the availability of guns is a major contribution to violence, and a handgun is the primary weapon used in 65 percent of homicides. It is 167 times more likely to be used in suicide than to kill a home intruder, 21 times more likely to kill a member of the family during a disagreement, and 6 times more likely to be involved in an accidental death. A loaded gun at home is even more likely (100 times) to kill a family member or friend than a burglar.

426. The answer is C. *(Hamburg, pp 128–134.)* Motor vehicle accidents are the major cause of death among adolescents and young adults. Physicians consider them to be of epidemic proportion among adolescents—in whom they account for 36 percent of all deaths. Homicide is the second leading cause of death; 25 percent of homicides occur in those 15 to 24 years old. Suicide is the third leading cause of death and is increasing for this age group, while it is decreasing for the general population. Infections and illicit drug abuse account for a relatively small number of deaths in this age group.

427. The answer is D. *(Lindzey, 3/e, pp 809–810.)* Social context and peer pressure are most important both in acquiring a habit of substance abuse and in maintaining it. The social context has been shown to be of primary importance in maintaining a habit of substance abuse, even for addicted heroin users. Substance abuse includes such addictive behaviors as smoking, drug abuse, and alcohol abuse. Peer pressure is especially effective with teenagers in initiating, terminating, and avoiding substance abuse, especially with cigarette smoking. The percentage of teenage smokers is still increasing, especially among teenage females. Attempts by such pioneers as Richard Evans to use peer pressure through social inoculation to prevent smoking among teenagers have been relatively effective. Becoming a teenage smoker has some immediate value, such as being accepted by one's peers, feeling more mature or adult, and defying authority figures. Arousal of fear and traditional methods of health education have had very limited effects on smoking and other addictive behaviors.

428. The answer is D. *(Kaplan, 7/e, pp 200, 753–756.)* Thomas Holmes and Richard Rahe developed a social readjustment rating scale that includes 43 life events that can cause varying amounts of stress and disruption in the lives of normal people (e.g., death of a spouse, separation or divorce, death of a close friend, changing or losing one's job, moving to a new location, retirement). Each stressful life event was assigned a unit score. They found that if one accumulated a certain number of stress or life-change units in a single year, the vulnerability to and incidence of psychosomatic disorders increased. Recent data show that persons who face these life-event readjustments optimistically rather than pessimistically are less apt to develop psychosomatic disorders or will recover from them more rapidly. The mechanism is still being explored, but a series of life-change events and a person's coping skills, values, and personality may combine to generate or "drive" physiologic correlates to influence genetically predisposed or vulnerable persons to develop a psychosomatic disorder. The Holmes and Rahe scale is being revised to incorporate the variability of individual values and social and physical status.

Friedman and Rosenman defined type A and type B personalities and developed a structured interview to identify the specific personal components in a type A or type B person. The Luria-Nebraska neuropsychological battery assesses a wide range of cognitive functions, e.g., dyslexia and dyscalculia, in addition to brain dysfunction and the localization of various cortical zones. The Minnesota multiphasic personality inventory (MMPI) is an objective, self-report test for assessing personality, and the Rorschach is a projective test originally designed to identify patterns of thinking and association and particularly various thought disorders.

429. The answer is D. *(Gatchel, 2/e, p 139.)* The human immunodeficiency virus (HIV) affects the immune system by decreasing T lymphocytes, some types of immunoglobulins, T-helper lymphocytes, and lymphocyte responsiveness to antigens, thus disrupting cellular immunity and increasing susceptibility to opportunistic infections. HIV is spread primarily through exchange of body fluids during sex, the sharing of needles or other drug paraphernalia, blood transfusion, and perinatal contact of an infected mother with her infant. Spread through fomites has not been documented. Other intimate exchanges of body fluids have been implicated but not yet documented, except in cases of contact with open lesions. While fairly rare, infections of health care workers with HIV by accidents with contaminated needles and blood have been documented.

430. The answer is A. *(Isselbacher, 13/e, p 2341.)* Fetal alcohol syndrome is a danger in those women who drink heavily during pregnancy. It is characterized by certain morphological abnormalities and is frequently associated with mental retardation. Fetal alcohol syndrome occurs in about 1 per 700 live births, which is more frequent than Down's syndrome (1 per 1000). The severity of the disorder is dose-related. Even two drinks daily of alcohol during pregnancy can also result in significantly decreased birth weight, and consumption levels as low as two drinks twice a week can increase the spontaneous abortion rate. Other adverse effects of alcohol consumption during pregnancy are attention-deficit disorder, lowered viability at birth, abnormalities of heart rate, poor sucking ability, and other behaviors associated with poor functioning of the central nervous system. Cigarette smoking combined with alcohol consumption during pregnancy results in an increased and potentiated risk.

431. The answer is E. *(Hamburg, pp 130–132.)* Among adolescents, the mortality is higher for males than for females. Motor vehicle accidents are the leading cause of death among males, followed by suicide and homicide. Accidents are linked with affluence and frequently related to alcohol consumption. Among females, especially those below the age of 18, the leading causes of death are complications of pregnancy, childbirth, and the puerperium.

432. The answer is E. *(Gatchel, 2/e, pp 114–119.)* Fifteen percent of the population (more than 35 million people) in the United States have hypertension. Risk factors for hypertension constitute complex interactions between behavioral, physiologic, and genetic factors. Age, race, and family history have been the standard risk factors, but they are not modifiable. More recently behavioral and environmental factors have been documented to play a significant role in the pathogenesis of hypertension. Of these behavioral risk factors, eating behaviors related to high intake of dietary salt and obesity are most relevant, followed by stress and personality factors, which are again related to a person's coping mechanisms. The complex interaction of these behavioral factors over time is most significant. Compliance with medical treatment is crucial after hypertension has developed, but not in its pathogenesis.

433. The answer is A. *(Isselbacher, 13/e, pp 1366–1371.)* Duodenal ulcer is chronic and recurrent in 6 to 15 percent of the population. It can also exist with or without symptoms. Hence, it is difficult to establish biologic and behavioral etiologies. Formerly, a personality exhibiting oral-receptive characteristics and unmet oral needs was thought to be a dominant causative factor, but such a personality designation has not been substantiated. Psychosocial and behavioral factors—particularly chronic anxiety, psychological stress, cigarette smoking, and diet (including alcohol and coffee)—do play a role in the exacerbation of ulcer activity. No difference in frequency of duodenal ulcers has been identified among different socioeconomic classes or occupation groups.

434. The answer is E. *(Isselbacher, 13/e, p 2341.)* Fetal alcohol syndrome can occur as the result of chronic heavy drinking by a pregnant woman. Symptoms may include severe retardation of intrauterine growth, premature birth, microcephaly, and other deformities such as congenital eye and ear problems, heart defects, extra fingers and toes, and patterns of disturbed sleep. It is the most prevalent cause of defective cerebral development. Most recent research suggests a 10 percent risk of this syndrome if the pregnant woman drinks as little as 2 to 4 ounces of hard liquor daily. It is estimated that 6000 infants a year suffer from the effects of fetal alcohol syndrome.

435. The answer is E. *(Hamburg, pp 140–141.)* Health-damaging behaviors of adolescents are very complex and involve some underlying influences and motivations that can be termed *risk factors* for problem behaviors. In general, these risk factors can be categorized as personal or personality factors, social or interpersonal factors, and cultural or environmental factors. While social or interpersonal and cultural or environmental factors are extremely important in understanding or predicting health-damaging behaviors, the personal and personality factors underlie the cognitive and emotional perceptions and reactions of each adolescent's behavior. The major personal or personality factors that underlie and influence the risk factors for problem behaviors are unconventionality, rebelliousness, high risk-taking behavior, a low value on achievement in both school and job performance, and a high value on being or attempting to appear autonomous.

436. The answer is B. *(Gatchel, 2/e, pp 281–289.)* Smoking is a behavior determined by multiple factors; however, a number of environmental factors have been found to place individual adolescents at greater risk of becoming regular smokers. Adolescents employed outside the home are more apt to start smoking (females having twice the risk); if both of their parents smoke they have twice the risk—less if one parent smokes; the greater the number of friends who smoke, the greater risk, especially if one's best friend smokes; adult role models (teachers, television stars, adult friends) who smoke increase the risk of the teenager's smoking. Positive-image and action-oriented advertising also increases the risk, as well as individual rebelliousness, not participating in organized school and community activities, low school achievement, impatience in assuming an adult role, and need for a sense of identity.

437. The answer is E. *(Gatchel, 2/e, pp 139–142.)* AIDS did not spread initially among college students, but they are now considered increasingly to be at risk. College students feel that the campus is a protected environment; however, they are at risk because of their frequent sexual contact. Also, they are less apt to practice "safe sex" because they still have a sense of invulnerability that was characteristic of their adolescence and because of their belief that their partners will let others know if they have AIDS. Some also believe that only homosexuals and drug users get AIDS. They need to know that AIDS cuts across all educational levels and that educated people do get AIDS. Some studies show that college students already have the knowledge about risks, but that their beliefs in the safety of the campus, in their student colleagues, and in their own invulnerability prevent them from practicing safe behavior.

438. The answer is D. *(Kandel, 3/e, p 806.)* A recent study showed that emotional problems were the cause of 70 percent of the cases of insomnia. Depression, which is characterized by early-morning awakening, was the most frequent cause of insomnia. Anxiety, positively correlated with difficulty in falling asleep, was also a frequent cause of insomnia. The most frequent presenting complaint was insomnia, not depression, and hence the problem was often treated initially with sleeping pills. The perception of insomnia is self-reported and can be quite independent of the actual number of hours slept. One study of 127 insomniacs observed a sleep duration of 7 h. Physiologic events (e.g., leg twitches, restless leg syndrome) do keep about 30 percent of insomniacs awake. Most insomniacs maintain higher core body temperatures during sleep, perhaps associated with an autonomic hyperarousal on a decreased deep slow-wave sleep. Anticipation of poor sleep can also cause insomnia (about 15 percent of cases).

439. The answer is D. *(Gatchel, 2/e, pp 71–73.)* Inability to cope with psychological stress has a direct physiologic effect and over time can cause damage to most systems of the body. The most frequently cited illnesses related to failure to cope with stress include coronary artery disease, hypertension, and gastrointestinal problems. Coping style and life-style are very important since they help determine the reaction to stress and they lead people to adopt behaviors and habits that can predispose them to illness. Cancer can be aggravated by psychological stress but the initial pathogenesis appears to be more dependent on other factors. Stress is increasingly considered to be a major factor in the prognosis of cancer.

440. The answer is D. *(Last, 13/e, pp 741–760.)* Research findings on the use of alcoholic beverages show that the life span of an alcoholic is on the average shortened by 10 to 12 years. Alcohol is considered to be a contributory cause in half of all deaths resulting from automobile accidents. The current rate of use of alcohol is estimated to be 70 to 90 percent. Recent research on the behavior and educational treatment of problem drinking and alcoholism has shown that total and permanent abstinence is no longer considered the only treatment objective. The total abstinence treatment was based on the belief that alcoholism is a physical disease characterized by craving for alcohol and loss of control over drinking during periods of intoxication. The disease model justified abstinence because one cannot allow a sick person to have access to the agent that causes the sickness. Abstinence was also an exquisitely simple treatment goal to define and monitor. Although total abstinence is appropriate in some instances, more recent empirical studies of the drinking behavior of alcoholics support the use of the social learning model for selected individuals. Various behavioral therapies are employed, such as the use of rewards rather than punishments and the pursuit of controlled social drinking rather than total abstinence as a therapy goal. The degree of addiction and dependence on alcohol is an important underlying factor. Heritability must also be assessed. The usual response of health policy makers and governments to alcohol-related health problems has been to think only in terms of increasing treatment services, which leaves the root causes essentially unaddressed. One of these root public policy issues is the complicated number of conflicting policies. Unlimited treatment facilities and services would be beyond all financial resources and still would not deal with the biologic, psychosocial, cultural, religious, and legal issues. An important first move may be to recommend that the goal for alcohol consumption be reduced to 2 gallons per person per year (from 2.54 gallons in 1987) as proclaimed as a health objective for the U.S. by the year 2000.

441. The answer is C. *(Gatchel, 2/e, pp 127–138.)* Bereavement from the loss of a loved one has been found to reduce the responsiveness of lymphocytes to mitogens. The same reaction occurs as a result of certain life-style factors, such as cigarette smoking and alcohol consumption. Psychological and social stress not only suppresses the immune system, but also suppresses DNA synthesis and DNA repair. Lack of close personal or family ties has been associated with reduced immune competence and with tumor growth. Environmental, physiologic, and psychosocial factors are thought to trigger the development and growth of cancer by suppressing the "surveillance" function of the immune system, which protects the body from invasion of alien cells and viruses. Exercise improves normal bodily functions, so the usual defense mechanisms should help protect against rather than enhance tumor growth.

442. The answer is E. *(Last, 13/e, pp 701–711.)* Research studies of behavior in illness and relationships with medical professionals clearly show the need for increased competency of the patient in adapting to and coping with conditions of illness and injury. This runs counter to the frequent appearance of dependency of the patient on the physician to manage and prevent an illness. Thus, the largest potential for promoting health will result from social action directed to the development of more healthful patterns of living, rather than increased use of physician services. Eliminating risk factors and attempting to modify patterns of behavior are important strategies for improving the health status of specific population groups.

443. The answer is E. *(Last, 13/e, pp 687–697.)* The major causes of death, serious illness, and disability in the United States today are chronic disease and violence. Chronic diseases account for 75 to 80 percent of all deaths. Accidents, suicide, and homicide account for another 10 percent. Another measure of the relative impact of various diseases and lethal forces is the concept of "potential years of life lost," which highlights the loss to society as a result of youthful or early death. The most recent life expectancy tables indicate that three categories—diseases of the circulatory system, cancer, and accidents and violence—account for about 72 percent of the potential years of life lost in the United States. Two chronic disease categories—diseases of the circulatory and musculoskeletal system—account for 38 percent of conditions causing disability and limitations of major activity. Behind most chronic diseases, disabilities, and premature deaths are many environmental and behavioral factors that are potentially amenable to change or prevention. Although the etiology is usually multidimensional, it is now recognized that environmental threats and individual behavior play a major role. It is estimated that about 80 percent of all cancer among men and 75 percent among women is attributable to environmental or behavioral factors or a combination of both. This percentage represents a great potential for prevention. The individual and societal life-style patterns and behaviors that constitute the major behavioral risk factors involved in chronic disease and severe disability include cigarette smoking, alcohol and other drug abuse, poor nutrition, lack of adequate physical activity, irresponsible use of motor vehicles, irresponsible use of guns and other manifestations of violence, the apparent decline of family health and social supports, sexual promiscuity or carelessness about contraception, and excessive television viewing. Information alone is insufficient for change, so health education must be directed at devising the most effective strategies for changing and then maintaining the individual and group behavior that promotes health and prevents disease. In spite of the apparent simplicity with which behavior is sometimes regarded, it is nevertheless one of the most difficult attributes of human beings to change, and one of the most complex issues is attempting to understand the biopsychosocial components and mechanisms of behavior. Yet most behavior is learned, and if something can be learned, then it should be possible to unlearn it and substitute and practice a more health-promoting behavior. A component of behavioral change that is often ignored is the environmental context under which a specific behavior is learned, the environmental context that maintains the behavior, and the changes that must be made in the environmental context if the behavior is going to be changed. Behavioral and risk profiles are important, but so is the environmental context within which a person lives.

444. The answer is E. *(Last, 13/e, pp 715–728.)* Intensive scientific studies begun in the 1940s have clearly established the health hazards associated with the use of tobacco products, particularly cigarettes. The overall mortality risk for smokers compared with nonsmokers is 60 percent greater. Each cigarette smoked shortens the smoker's life span by at least 5.5 min. Studies in the 1950s showed that smokers were much more likely than nonsmokers to die from a large number of diseases. Lung cancer, cardiovascular disease, and emphysema are three of the more significant diseases associated with smoking. The risk of dying of lung cancer, for example, is between 8 and 15 times higher in cigarette smokers than in nonsmokers. More recent studies have led to the realization that there is a serious impact of smoking pollution on the health of nonsmokers. For example, children whose parents smoke have a higher incidence of respiratory infections and impaired function than those whose parents do not smoke. In 1989 there were 142,000 deaths from lung cancer with 83 percent attributed to smoking. More women than men are initiating smoking and the rate of mortality for women is increasing more rapidly than for men. In 1985, smoking initiating rates were 34.6 percent for women and 33.4 percent for men, and fewer women (39.8 percent) were quitting than men (49 percent).

445. The answer is D. *(Isselbacher, 13/e, pp 446–452.)* Maintaining a lean body is conducive to good health and a long life. Actuarial studies have shown that obesity is associated with a diminished life expectancy. A 50-year-old man who is 50 pounds overweight has half the remaining life expectancy of a normal-weight man of the same age. Excess weight can aggravate existing health problems, causing more severe symptoms or accelerating the appearance of a disorder earlier in life than might otherwise occur. Experts in heart disease estimate that at least one-fourth of our problems with cardiovascular disease are attributable to obesity, which makes the heart and lungs work harder than normal. Hypertension is twice as common among the obese as among lean persons. Although obesity is not the leading cause of hypertension, it does contribute to hypertension, which in turn can cause death from heart and kidney disease and stroke. Many people with high blood pressure are able to bring their pressure down to normal levels without drugs by losing weight and reducing their consumption of salt. Obesity also increases the risk of developing diabetes about fourfold and is associated with heart disease, blood clots, varicose veins, gout, respiratory disease, gastrointestinal disorders, gallbladder and liver disease, and arthritis of weight-bearing joints. Overweight people appear to be more clumsy, react to unexpected events more slowly, and are more likely to have accidents than normal-weight people. Compared with the general population, overweight people are more likely to die in automobile accidents. They have also been shown to be more susceptible to complications of surgery, infections, and delayed healing of wounds.

446. The answer is A. *(Rosen, p 112.)* There are many claims of health benefits from exercise, but the greatest scientific evidence supports the prevention of coronary heart disease, the maintenance of optimal body weight and body composition, and the normalization of fat and carbohydrate metabolism. There is also good support for the prevention of hypertension, osteoporosis, and low back pain and for improved psychological status. While exercise has not been shown to prevent such diseases as type I diabetes, chronic obstructive lung disease, renal failure, or arthritis, it has been shown to result in clinical improvement of these and other diseases after they have become manifest.

447. The answer is D. *(Rosen, pp 117–118.)* Exercise has a major effect on the amount of fat in relation to lean tissue and body weight. Exercise of moderate intensity can result in an increase in energy expenditure of 300 kcal for 30 min of activity. Also the metabolic rate remains elevated for several hours after physical activity, which further increases the contribution of exercise to weight loss. Exercise is important in the elderly as it helps retain muscle mass. Exercise also contributes to general weight loss, especially when combined with calorie restriction, as it causes a greater proportion of weight loss to be from adipose tissue.

448. The answer is E. *(Last, 13/e, pp 967–968, 986.)* Down's syndrome (mongolism) is caused by a chromosomal aberration. Most sufferers have 47 chromosomes instead of 46. The risk of Down's syndrome increases dramatically with maternal age, especially after age 35. The general incidence is about 1:700 live births, varying from about 1:2000 live births in early childbearing age to about 1:400 at age 35 and about 1:100 at age 40. About 80 percent of Down's syndrome infants will have standard trisomy, about 15 percent will have the translocation form, and 5 percent will have the mosaic form. About one-third of the translocation cases are inherited and detectable in one or the other parent. Aminocentesis can detect the presence of Down's syndrome, but the procedure requires surgical skill, is not free from hazard, and, if the test is positive, introduces ethical and religious considerations of potential induced abortion. Down's syndrome accounts for about 30 percent of the retarded children in the United States. Although some sufferers have a relatively normal IQ, most IQs are between 40 and 60. Most children used to die early, but with antibiotics and other scientific advances, those who live to the preschool age can now be expected to live to the average age of 40.

449. The answer is E. *(Gatchel, 2/e, pp 105–111.)* Most of the characteristic risk factors for cardiovascular disease are behavioral. The usual factors of hypertension, cholesterolemia, and cigarette smoking have basic behavioral bases, particularly in terms of stress, diet, and behavioral addictions, but others such as obesity, personality type, and physical inactivity are also behaviorally based. Advanced age, male sex, and diabetes are less behaviorally related (but still have behavioral components). A high concentration of glucose without overt diabetes is both behaviorally (via diet) and metabolically related. A small amount of alcohol consumption appears to decrease risk, but excessive amounts increase risk, especially when combined with smoking behavior and type A personality.

450. The answer is D. *(Gatchel, 2/e, pp 114–119.)* One of the earliest psychosocial hypotheses in the etiology of hypertension was that it was anger directed inward because of an inability to express anger properly. While it has been demonstrated that hypertensive persons do tend to avoid involvement and confrontation, additional relevant factors are involved. Acutely stressful events have been related to hypertension, and it has been demonstrated that persons with a familial history of hypertension have an increased response to environmental and behavioral stressors compared with normotensive controls. Increased sympathetic nervous system activity and diminished parasympathetic inhibition result in increased blood pressure, which suggests a possible disturbance of central autonomic regulation with possible increased sensitivity to stressors.

451. The answer is D. *(Gatchel, 2/e, pp 282–289.)* Cigarette smoking is a powerful addiction; it is estimated that about 60 percent of smokers have tried to quit and another 30 percent want to quit. While nicotine may be the major pharmacologic reinforcer and behavioral factors play a role in the reinforcement of the addiction, behavioral factors have been demonstrated to play a major role in the initiation of the smoking habit itself, the day-to-day fluctuations in smoking, and the difficulty of maintaining abstinence after one has quit. Behavioral factors also play a major role in the situations in which smoking occurs and in the choice of cigarette brands. Of the estimated 30 million smokers who try to quit each year, only about 3 million achieve long-term abstinence. A physician's advice has a low 1-year abstinence result, except for patients recovering from a recent heart attack, in whom the 1-year abstinence is about 50 percent.

452. The answer is B. *(Isselbacher, 13/e, pp 2414–2419.)* Twin, family, and adoptive studies have shown that schizophrenia has a significant and primary genetic basis. Even though psychosocial factors are regarded as secondary, the stress-diathesis model incorporates a host of stressful factors that may precipitate a psychotic state in a person at high risk. The stress can be the result of specific illnesses, social or psychological, environmental, or chemical (such as that from use of PCP or amphetamines). Also, specific hallucinogens may precipitate a psychotic episode that is indistinguishable from schizophrenia. There is no specific schizophrenia-prone personality type, even though a small percentage of persons with a schizoid and paranoid personality disorder seem to be more vulnerable to developing schizophrenic disorders. Lower socioeconomic status does correlate with a higher incidence of schizophrenia. The onset of schizophrenia is generally related to a developmental or intrapsychic deficit in the vulnerable individual.

Health Care Systems

DIRECTIONS: Each question below contains five suggested responses. Select the **one best** response to each question.

453. Patients seek the services of "nonscientific," in preference to "scientific," systems of healing primarily because these services are

(A) less costly
(B) more available
(C) more efficacious
(D) more supportive
(E) none of the above

454. Which of the following health professions had the highest percentage of women enrolled in 1991?

(A) Medicine
(B) Dentistry
(C) Pharmacy
(D) Optometry
(E) Veterinary medicine

455. The statistics for 1990 show that intravenous drug users accounted for what percentage of the infections with human immunodeficiency virus (HIV) among men?

(A) 3
(B) 13
(C) 23
(D) 33
(E) 43

456. Long-term care for elderly widowed parents is most often provided by

(A) health professional caregivers
(B) nursing homes
(C) sisters or brothers
(D) daughters
(E) long-time friends

457. The folk medical care system employed by many Mexicans and Mexican-Americans is known as

(A) *medico*
(B) allopathy
(C) voodoo
(D) soma
(E) *curanderismo*

458. The form of treatment that most resembles *curanderismo* in its techniques of therapy is

(A) allopathy
(B) homeopathy
(C) osteopathy
(D) chiropractic
(E) spiritual healing

459. In the United States since 1900,

(A) cancer deaths have increased 50 percent
(B) gastrointestinal infections have increased
(C) life expectancy for both men and women has increased by 50 percent
(D) heart disease has been reduced to pre-1900 levels
(E) the number of AIDS cases reached a peak in 1989 and leveled off

460. International statistics on the per capita consumption of absolute alcohol in liters show which country to rate the highest?

(A) Finland
(B) United States
(C) Russia
(D) Spain
(E) France

461. Between 1950 and 1985, the greatest total percentage increase in per capita consumption of alcoholic beverages was in

(A) Finland
(B) France
(C) the former German Democratic Republic (East Germany)
(D) Netherlands
(E) United States

462. Medicare expenditures are correctly characterized by which of the following statements?

(A) Ten percent of Medicare enrollees account for over 70 percent of all Medicare expenditures
(B) Over 50 percent of Medicare expenditures are for care in the last year of life
(C) Fifteen percent of all Medicare enrollees have no reimbursable expenses in a given year
(D) Only 5 percent of Medicare enrollees over age 85 have no reimbursable Medicare expenses
(E) The 6 percent of Medicare patients who die each year consume over 50 percent of all Medicare expenses

463. True statements regarding the deinstitutionalization of patients in state mental hospitals since 1955 include which of the following?

(A) It has been attributed to the improved treatment (drug) programs in state mental hospitals

(B) It provided a last resort for one class of society's rejected mentally ill population

(C) It resulted in an initially decreased public investment in mental health and a subsequent increase in the 1980s

(D) It resulted in local, state, and federal agencies taking comprehensive responsibility for psychiatric and social services for the chronically mentally ill

(E) Both private and public hospitals are now required to take severely mentally ill patients without insurance

464. During the early and mid-1980s the number of

(A) registered nurses (RNs) decreased

(B) physician assistants (PAs) decreased

(C) midwives increased

(D) licensed practical nurses (LPNs) increased

(E) nurse practitioners (NPs) decreased

DIRECTIONS: Each numbered question or incomplete statement below is NEGATIVELY phrased. Select the **one best** lettered response.

465. Native-American healers are responsible for discovering and using all the following EXCEPT

(A) the cure for scurvy
(B) oral contraception
(C) the use of antibiotics
(D) nearly 50 drugs now officially listed in the *National Formulary*
(E) an appreciation of the integration of humans and nature

466. A health maintenance organization is characterized by all the following key principles EXCEPT

(A) provision of comprehensive medical care to its enrolled members
(B) emphasis on efficiency and economy as well as medical care
(C) strong emphasis on preventive health services
(D) members who pay only for the services received
(E) reduction of time spent in the hospital

467. Correct characterizations of the elderly in the health care system include all the following EXCEPT

(A) 15 to 20 percent of the noninstitutionalized elderly have limitations in activities of daily living
(B) 5 percent of the elderly reside in nursing homes or institutions
(C) only 15 percent of the functionally limited elderly are receiving needed help from the formal medical or nonfamily system
(D) most elderly initially consult a health care provider in a health crisis
(E) there are twice as many disabled elderly being cared for by their families as by institutions

468. The Patient Self-Determination Act allows a patient to do all the following EXCEPT

(A) refuse medical care
(B) specify in advance procedures to which the patient will submit
(C) specify in advance procedures to which the patient will not submit
(D) specify in advance circumstances for which life-support technology will not be used
(E) designate a surrogate decision-maker who is subject to overrule only by the personal physician

469. True statements about the nursing profession include all the following EXCEPT

(A) nearly three-fourths of all working registered nurses are employed in hospitals and nursing homes
(B) only 80 percent of the potentially employable registered nurses in the United States are working full-time
(C) hospitals report a very high turnover rate, often as high as 50 percent of the nursing staff annually
(D) there are more than 1.5 million registered nurses in the United States
(E) nurses are the largest single group of health professionals in the United States

470. The principles of the hospice movement include all the following EXCEPT

(A) acceptance of death as a logical part of life
(B) self-determination
(C) importance of family support
(D) control of pain only when severe
(E) direction of services usually by the primary care physician

471. Studies of the economics of health care show that all the following statements are true EXCEPT

(A) between 1940 and 1990, the percentage of gross national product spent on health tripled
(B) per capita expenditures for health care increased nearly tenfold between 1950 and 1977
(C) government expenditures for health care have increased nearly 2000 percent since 1950
(D) current health expenditures by the federal government represent 13 percent of the total federal budget
(E) the federal government contributes 72 percent of the funds in the total health care field

472. Economic benefits of health promotion programs to the employer are seen in all the following areas EXCEPT

(A) company pension fund costs
(B) worker absenteeism
(C) worker morale
(D) life and disability insurance costs
(E) cessation of smoking

473. All the following statements about the early history of medical education in the United States are correct EXCEPT that

(A) the first medical school in the United States was established in 1783 at Harvard University

(B) the American Medical Association (AMA) at its founding in 1847 had as a primary goal the reform of medical education

(C) the Association of American Medical Colleges (AAMC) was organized in 1876 as part of the effort to improve the quality of medical education

(D) in 1902, the *Journal of the American Medical Association (JAMA)* began publishing medical school failure statistics on state licensing board examinations

(E) in 1905, only five medical schools required any college preparation for admission

474. All the following statements concerning health care for the elderly are true EXCEPT

(A) demands on the health care system are expected to increase for the over-65 age group

(B) acute diseases are expected to increase in all segments of the over-65 age group

(C) mortality among the elderly has shown a decline over the past 15 years

(D) the sex differential in human longevity is the cumulative result of excessive male mortality throughout the life span

(E) females have been the heaviest users of the health care system

DIRECTIONS: Each group of questions below consists of lettered headings followed by a set of numbered items. For each numbered item select the **one** lettered heading with which it is **most** closely associated. Each lettered heading may be used **once, more than once, or not at all.**

Questions 475–477

For each health care plan described, select the payment plan with which it is most closely associated.

(A) Medicare
(B) National health insurance
(C) Medicaid
(D) Blue Cross
(E) Blue Shield

475. A physician and hospital insurance plan whose cost is shared by employees and employers through Social Security payroll taxes

476. A prepayment insurance plan providing limited coverage of hospital costs on a nonprofit basis for individuals or groups

477. A grant-in-aid program whose costs are shared by the federal and state governments for all low-income persons

Questions 478–480

For each health care description, select the health care option in which it is included.

(A) Health maintenance organization (HMO)
(B) Fee-for-service system
(C) National health insurance program
(D) Managed care
(E) Preferred provider organization (PPO)

478. A competitive, cost-conscious, for-profit, integrated plan for financing and delivery of health care

479. A single-payer universal health care system

480. A contractual medical insurance arrangement between selected physicians, hospitals, and insurers

Questions 481–483

Match the descriptions below with the appropriate medical problem.

(A) Neoplasms
(B) Circulatory disorders
(C) Mental disorders
(D) Musculoskeletal disorders
(E) None of the above

481. The greatest number of Social Security disability awards for women

482. The greatest number of Social Security disability awards for men and women combined

483. The most rapidly increasing rate of Social Security disability awards

Questions 484–486

For each approximate percentage change in mortality between 1980 and 1991, select the cause of death with which it is associated.

(A) Disease of the heart
(B) Malignant neoplasm
(C) Chronic obstructive pulmonary disease
(D) Cerebrovascular disease
(E) Suicide

484. Increased by 1 percent

485. Increased by 26 percent

486. Decreased by 34 percent

Health Care Systems

Answers

453. The answer is D. *(Twaddle, 2/e, pp 155, 165–182.)* Although cost and availability may contribute to a patient's decision to seek "nonscientific" health care, the main attraction of such treatment is that it more often serves a patient's psychological needs than do "scientific" systems of health care. "Scientific" medicine frequently contradicts patients' cultural beliefs and expectations and ignores their psychological and social plight. The nontraditional system recognizes that healing also occurs within the intimate context of family, community, and religion.

454. The answer is C. *(U.S. Public Health Service, pp 5, 221.)* The number of women enrolled for training in the health professions has continued to increase over the past decade. Pharmacy has the highest with 63 percent, followed by veterinary medicine with 62.1 percent, optometry with 49.5 percent, and allopathic medicine with 38.1 percent. Dentistry has 35.9 percent women enrolled, followed by osteopathic medicine with 33.4 percent. Over the past decade, podiatry has shown the greatest increase, followed by optometry and dentistry. Veterinary medicine from 41.8 to 62.1 percent and pharmacy increased from 50.1 to 63 percent. Enrollment of women in medicine increased from 28 to 38 percent, and nursing has decreased from 94 to 90 percent women.

455. The answer is C. *(U.S. Public Health Service, pp 145–146.)* As of 1993, intravenous drug users accounted for 29.1 percent of the HIV cases among men. Men who are both intravenous drug users and homosexual accounted for an additional 6.3 percent of the HIV cases. Adult and adolescent homosexual and bisexual men accounted for 56.1 percent of the HIV cases. Among women with HIV, 49.2 percent acquired their infection through intravenous drug use. Heterosexual contact accounted for 33.2 percent of the HIV infections among women. As of 1990, approximately 87 percent of all HIV infections occurred among adult or adolescent men, 12 percent among adult or adolescent women, and 2 percent among children under 2 years of age. Increases are occurring in intravenous drug users and heterosexuals, as well as in total number of infections.

456. The answer is D. *(Hazzard, 3/e, pp 229–233.)* When elderly parents are widowed, most of the long-term care is given by their adult children, primarily by a daughter. Contrary to the modern myth, adult children are not alienated from their aged parents and they make strenuous efforts to avoid institutional placement of the elderly. These middle-generation women are under increasing stress, however, because their traditional roles as wives, homemakers, parents, grandparents, and parental caregivers are now being increasingly expanded as women join the labor force. Sixty percent of women between the ages of 45 and 54 are employed, and more than 40 percent of women between the ages of 55 and 64 are now employed. This remains an increasing trend.

457. The answer is E. *(Twaddle, 2/e, pp 175–176.)* Curanderismo is a very popular and widely used system of folk medicine. It is a blend of Native-American medicine, Mexican folk medicine, African folk medicine, and European medieval medicine. This health care system is an important source of cultural solidarity and pride for practitioner and client alike. Indeed, the social and cultural aspects of *curanderismo* may well overshadow the practical concerns of actually getting well.

458. The answer is D. *(Twaddle, 2/e, p 175.)* Curanderismo, like chiropractic, stresses manipulation and massage of body parts as a major part of its therapeutic technology. However, *curanderismo* also enlists the aid of various medicines and poultices, including mood-changing drugs. Manipulation and massage are important in helping to establish rapport between physician and patient. Indeed, the importance of "laying on" of hands is recognized by virtually all effective systems of the curative arts.

459. The answer is C. *(Gatchel, 2/e, pp 5–6.)* With the advent of vaccinations and antibiotics to treat and prevent infectious illnesses and with the changes in health care and health behavior practices, the life expectancy for both men and women has increased by 50 percent. The high incidence of death from diseases such as influenza, pneumonia, diphtheria, tuberculosis, and gastrointestinal infections has been reduced to less than 5 percent of 1900 levels. These infectious diseases have now been replaced by many other diseases caused by life-style and behavior. Increased numbers of deaths are now caused by or facilitated by preventable behavioral factors such as smoking, poor diet, substance abuse, lack of exercise, and stressful conditions. A reduction in heart disease has been made over the past few decades, but levels have not yet reached those of 1900. The number of AIDS cases has continued to increase over the past 15 years, with the greatest increases occurring in the heterosexual and adolescent populations.

460. The answer is E. *(Last, 13/e, pp 745–750.)* The highest per capita alcohol consumption by regions is in Australia and New Zealand, North America, and Europe. These regions are the most economically developed, share similar cultural heritages, and have a long history of acceptance and use of alcohol. France has the highest per capita consumption of alcohol (13.3 L) and Spain is third with 11.8 L per capita. The U.S. ranks sixteenth with 8.0 L per capita per year, Finland thirty-sixth with 6.9 L, and Russia fiftieth with 5.2 L per capita. Other countries with the highest per capita consumption include Barbados, Luxembourg, Argentina, and Portugal. In the past 10 years, France has shown a significant decrease in per capita consumption and seven other countries have shown a small decrease. This has been attributed to changes in some consuming populations, economic trends, recent efforts of governments to deal with alcohol problems, and an increased awareness of health-related risks.

461. The answer is C. *(Last, 13/e, pp 745–760.)* Since World War II, there has been a general trend of increased production and consumption of alcohol. Major per capita consumption increases have been recorded in Europe, North America, Australia, and New Zealand. The countries with the greatest per capita increases between 1950 and 1985 were the German Democratic Republic (758 percent), the Federal Republic of Germany (272 percent), the Netherlands (305 percent), Finland (282 percent), and Poland (133 percent). Other countries with over a 100 percent increase were Denmark, Hungary, and Czechoslovakia. The U.S. has shown a 60 percent increase while France has shown a 23 percent decrease. Of interest is that each of the top eight countries showing the greatest increase has increased at a faster rate each decade, while France, Austria, Portugal, Yugoslavia, Ireland, and Britain have experienced a slight decrease, especially since 1976. The World Health Organization has expressed concern that the conduct of international trade and marketing in alcoholic beverages constitutes a serious international public health problem.

462. The answer is A. *(Hazzard, 3/e, pp 167–175.)* The distribution of Medicare expenditures for those over age 65 is highly skewed, especially for care in a nursing home, less for hospital care, and less for physician and drug costs. This skewness is because only 10 percent of Medicare patients account for over 70 percent of all Medicare expenditures. On the other hand, it is important to recognize that about 35 percent of Medicare enrollees have no reimbursable expenses in any given year. Even 20 percent of persons over age 85 have no reimbursable expenses in a given year. The last year of life is often very expensive, so that the 6 percent of Medicare patients who die each year consume nearly 30 percent of all Medicare expenditures. Thus, a relatively small number of older persons consume the major portion of Medicare expenditures.

463. The answer is A. *(Last, 13/e, pp 956–958.) Deinstitutionalization* is a term used to describe the continuous decline in numbers of patients in state mental hospitals. It began about 1955 partly as the result of improved drug treatment programs. Policy and legislative changes 10 years later resulted in geographic decentralization and removed much of the power for involuntary commitments away from the mental hospitals (patients the hospitals had to accept). Thus, the state hospitals, which had provided a last resort for one class of society's rejected population (the chronically mentally ill), reduced their census and transferred much of the financial responsibility to the state and local communities. The public investment in mental health increased initially with federal funds supporting the decentralization. However, the federal support was gradually withdrawn during the 1980s and the state and local agencies have been unable to take responsibility for the comprehensive psychiatric and social services needed by the chronically mentally ill. Private hospitals treat more patients from the upper socioeconomic classes. Severely mentally ill patients without insurance generally are not accepted at private hospitals, so they must be admitted to public hospitals.

464. The answer is C. *(Williams, SJ, 3/e, pp 326–331.)* The number of registered nurses (RNs) has actually doubled over the past 30 years, so that by 1983 there were about 1.4 million employed licensed registered nurses. By 1986 the number of RNs had increased to 1.6 million. Yet a shortage remains because of the need for more personnel to operate new technology and to care for sicker patients. In addition, inferior wages and working conditions (short staffing, perceived lack of respect and authority) dissuade some prospective nurses. Licensed practical nurses (LPNs) have decreased from over 267,000 in 1982 to fewer than 205,000 in 1986. LPNs are assuming more and more duties in hospitals, but they have little upward mobility as RN nursing programs refuse to allow transfer credits. The number of physician assistants (PAs) has increased since their inception in 1966 to about 18,000 on 1985. About 75 percent work with physicians in primary care settings and others in internal medicine and surgery. Their number in hospitals is also increasing. Nurse-midwives have increased in number from 300 in the mid-1960s to 2700 certified nurse-midwives in 1983. Most work in hospitals and rural areas where they provide care for women who do not have private physicians, but a growing number are entering private practice, where they refer high-risk problems to physicians. In 1960, 83 percent of nursing graduates were trained in hospitals, but by 1980, 83 percent were trained in college and university programs. Nurse practitioners (NPs) are registered nurses who have completed advanced programs preparing them for expanded roles and responsibilities (e.g., health histories, physical examinations, formulating and managing care for acute and chronically ill patients). By 1980, there were about 16,000 NPs with 2000 additional graduates each year.

465. The answer is D. *(Twaddle, 2/e, pp 176–179.)* Native-American health care systems have contributed more to Western scientific medicine than any other cultural healing art. The ethnocentricity of Euro-Americans with respect to medicine has prevented our recognition and appreciation of this contribution. In so doing, we have ignored a large and important part of our cultural heritage. Native-American tribes discovered cures for scurvy, herbal oral contraception, the use of antibiotics, and more than 200 drugs that are now officially listed in the *United States Pharmacopeia* since its first edition in 1920. It is not generally realized that knowledge and other benefits did not flow exclusively from our scientific Western culture into the so-called lower cultures of Native-American civilizations. In fact, the advice of Native-American healers was much sought after by white patients and physicians alike. In addition to the herbs and healing techniques, Native-American healing systems relied heavily on a reverence for all forms of natural processes and were designed to preserve or reestablish the integration of humans and nature, i.e., harmony or balance between all living things and objects.

466. The answer is D. *(Williams, SJ, 3/e, pp 144–147.)* Physicians affiliated with health maintenance organizations (HMOs) have a strong financial incentive to provide medical care to enrolled members in a manner that emphasizes efficiency and economy. Prepayment for maintenance of health dictates minimal expenditures for patient care in order to maximize income. Means of accomplishing this include reducing the time patients spend in the hospital, doing as much diagnosis and therapy as possible on an outpatient basis, detecting disease early, and emphasizing preventive services. The HMOs have provided comprehensive services with greater economy and containment of costs than traditional fee-for-service arrangements.

467. The answer is D. *(Hazzard, 3/e pp 229–233.)* It is important to recognize that most of the elderly are able to function independently even though most have at least one chronic health condition. A survey by the U.S. Department of Health and Human Services found that 18 percent of the elderly population have limitations in activities of daily living, but only 5 percent of the elderly are residents of nursing homes or other institutions. Only 15 percent of the elderly with functional disabilities receive the help they need from the formal medical or nonfamily health care system. The vast majority of the elderly initially consult a relative or friend in a health crisis rather than a medical health care provider. There are twice as many elderly being cared for by their families as are being cared for by institutions. Daughters, and in some cases daughters-in-law, are the principal caregivers in the family. This will become an increasing problem with the increase of middle-aged women in the work force.

468. The answer is E. *(Sierles, pp 171–172.)* The Patient Self-Determination Act was passed by Congress in 1990 and became effective December 1, 1991. It guarantees a patient the right to refuse medical care, to specify advance directives (the measures or procedures a patient would want or would refuse under a variety of potential circumstances), and to specify an individual who would have the authority to make medical decisions (durable power of attorney) if the patient was unable to do so. Thus, a patient could specify that a breathing respirator or even cardiopulmonary resuscitation (CPR) not be used in an emergency. Possible circumstances can be specified (e.g., irreversible coma) for which the patient wants no intervention through medical technology.

469. The answer is B. *(Williams, SJ, 3/e, pp 326–332.)* There are more than 5 million people employed in health-related occupations. One-half of these are in nursing or related services, and they constitute the largest single group of health professionals in the country. Nursing remains a largely hospital-based profession. Nearly 75 percent of all nurses employed work in hospitals and nursing homes, and only 13 percent work in private physicians' offices and similar work places. The number of registered nurses in practice has grown since 1977, when it was 978,000, to 1,404,000 in 1983. Many hospitals report very high turnover rates in their nursing staffs. A rate of 50 percent turnover in a year is not unusual for many community and teaching hospitals in the United States. With more than 1.5 million registered nurses in the United States, less than half of the employable nurses are working full-time. Increased demand will come from acute-care hospitals, long-term care, home-based care, and preventive care. Also, the nursing profession has been attempting to increase and enhance its role and responsibility, especially over the past 2 decades.

470. The answer is E. *(Hazzard, 3/e, pp 383–385.)* The hospice movement is an attempt to provide care for the dying person progressing along the journey of life toward death. It deals with some of the major psychological and social conflicts encountered by patient, family, and health care provider when patients are dying. The basic principles of the movement are self-determination, acceptance of death as a logical part of life, and the importance of family support. These are accomplished through providing inpatient, outpatient, and home services under the direction of the primary care physicians; using the concept of the health care team; providing most primary care roles through family, hospice staff, and volunteers; early control of symptoms through aggressive and innovative approaches to pain, fear, and stress; support for family before and after patient's death; and support for the staff and caregivers. Most often the patient is kept at home and as comfortable as possible until death.

471. The answer is E. *(Sierles, pp 439–455.)* Health care costs in the United States are increasing at an alarming rate, with health expenditures representing an increasingly larger portion of family and governmental budgets. Current health expenditures by the federal government represent 13 percent of the total federal budget, with the federal budget containing 40 percent of the funds for all health costs. Between 1940 and 1990 the percentage of GNP spent on health care tripled from 4.1 to 12.7 percent. Per capita expenditures for health care increased from $78 in 1950 to $1365 in 1980. The causes of the rise in health care costs are multiple. General inflation has contributed to this to some extent, but other factors include the dramatic shift in the federal government's role of providing third-party payment for significant segments of the population and the increases in technology and subspecialization, litigation, drug use, and for-profit insurance and other services. As these costs increase without apparent limit, legislators and other public officials are looking increasingly to prevention, in general, and life-style change, in particular, to bring these cost increases under control.

472. The answer is A. *(Rosen, pp 239–247.)* Recent analyses of the economic benefits of most health promotion programs in the work place show benefits in such areas as savings through smoking-cessation programs, less worker absenteeism, improved worker attitude and morale, decreased life and disability insurance costs, less use of medical care services, and increased recruitment value. All of these savings, however, appear to be overshadowed by the increased costs and demands on the company's pension fund. In effect, the prevention programs would prolong the lives of former workers in their economically nonproductive years. The question being debated by employers now is who will pay for the longer and better lives of the workers.

473. The answer is A. *(Last, 13/e, pp 1065–1073.)* Today's physician receives vastly different training from the practitioner in eighteenth- or nineteenth-century America. Today's medical practitioner has pursued a rigorous course of study in clinical practice under the close supervision of faculty who are typically at the forefront of the field of academic medicine. In colonial America, there were very few physicians. The first medical school was established in 1756 at the College of Philadelphia (later, University of Pennsylvania). The second school was founded at King's College (later, Columbia University) in 1768. At the time of the Revolutionary War, there were estimated to be 3500 practitioners in the colonies of which only 400 had received any formal training. Apprenticeship to a practicing physician was the most common approach to training for a long period of time. The American Medical Association was founded in 1847 with the reform of medical education as a primary goal. In 1876, 22 medical schools organized the Association of American

Medical Colleges as part of an effort to improve the quality of medical education. Beginning in 1902, *JAMA* published medical school failure statistics on state board licensing examinations, a form of exposure that could not help but embarrass and lead to institutional reform. In 1905, only five schools required any college preparation for admission. Ten years later, 85 schools prescribed a minimum of 1 to 2 years of college preparation. By 1932, every recognized medical school and most of the state licensing boards required at least 2 years of college work. Many required 3 years, and several required a college degree.

474. The answer is B. *(Hazzard, 3/e pp 167–175.)* The elderly use a disproportionate amount of health care resources. With the estimated increase in the 65-and-over age group from 24 million (11 percent) to 38 million (14 percent), there will be an increased demand for health care services between now and the year 2000. Also, with the shift of health problems from acute illness to more chronic and debilitating conditions, there will be additional need to increase continuing and long-term health care. Data show women to be heavier users for services than men. With the increase in the elderly and with the female population progressively outnumbering the male population, the need for health care and help with social and economic problems in elderly females is expected to increase. The greater part of the sex differential in human longevity is considered to be the cumulative result of excessive male mortality throughout the life span. This is because of increased risk behaviors and habits that increase the vulnerability of males to health problems. The decline in mortality of the elderly over the past 15 years is partly due to the reduction in mortality from cardiovascular disease, improvements in medical science, and a shift in the population toward gathering more information and having more concern about their own health behaviors.

475–477. The answers are 475-A, 476-D, 477-C. *(Sierles, pp 439–455.)* Medicare has two basic components. Part A is a compulsory hospital insurance plan for persons 65 years or older who are entitled to benefits under the Social Security or Railroad Retirement Acts. Social Security payroll taxes provide the funds for inpatient diagnostic studies, hospital room and board costs, and some home care and extended care services. Part B is a voluntary supplementary insurance program that pays for a major part of outpatient visits, diagnostic studies, doctors' fees, home health services, and certain medical equipment. Costs are shared between the individual and the Federal General Revenue Fund, except for a deductible charge that is steadily increasing.

Blue Cross is a prepaid, limited "nonprofit" commercial medical insurance plan to cover hospital costs. It has grown rapidly with the burgeoning costs of hospital care. It also has become increasingly burdensome as a negotiated health care benefit between industry and labor.

Blue Shield is the same kind of payment mechanism as Blue Cross, extended to cover physicians' fees in hospitals as well as surgery and emergency care. Blue Cross, Blue Shield, Medicare, and Medicaid reimburse physicians and hospitals on a "reasonable cost" basis, which has continued to increase dramatically, and limit the decision-making responsibilities and authority of physicians and hospitals. Blue Cross and Blue Shield administer about 50 percent of private coverage.

The federal and state governments share the costs of Medicaid, although the program is administered by the states. The program provides medical care for low-income people of all ages and can complement some of the provisions of Medicare if the patient is without funds and if the health care provider will accept Medicaid patients. Medicare and Medicaid are providing limited and decreasing care. In spite of the four major payment plans discussed above, the major problems of equity, effectiveness, and economy still exist and are worsening. A very large segment of the population has no medical insurance coverage.

There is no national health insurance program at the present time. With the increasing number of citizens with no health insurance or affordable health care, and the constantly increasing costs of health care, health technology, and commercial insurance, there have been strong political pressures toward a national health insurance or single-payer health care system available to all citizens, but these have been countered by even stronger commercial pressures.

478–480. The answers are 478-D, 479-C, 480-E. *(Sierles, pp 439–455.)* Managed care is a competitive, integrated, cost-conscious, for-profit plan for financing and delivering medical care. It emerged from the 1973 HMO Act and offers selected providers of comprehensive care, programs for quality assurance and utilization review, and financial incentives for members to use selected providers and for physicians to practice cost-conscious medicine. The managed care plans have attempted to combine some of the benefits of PPOs and HMOs, but rely more heavily on cost-conscious reimbursement systems and competition.

A national health insurance program, or single-payer program, would be similar to the Canadian health care system with its universal coverage. Patients would select their own physicians and receive appropriate health care, and providers would be paid by a single-payer (the government or an insurance group) using a set schedule or per-capita basis. Costs would be significantly reduced through lower administrative costs and profits, an annually negotiated set of fees, and prevention measures. Insurance would not depend on employment status. Services would be provided on the basis of patient need and allocation of resources.

A health maintenance organization (HMO) is a prepaid health plan. It combines insurance coverage with health care delivery to an individual, and payment is based on a set monthly fee or capitation per enrollee. With a few fixed by contract, there is a strong incentive to promote wellness, which should result in fewer visits, lower costs, and higher profits, depending in part on whether the HMO is a nonprofit or for-profit organization. Most physicians are full-time and salaried.

A preferred provider organization (PPO) is primarily a contractual arrangement between individual physicians and hospitals and an insurance carrier or employer. The insurance company or employer negotiates lower prices for the services, and the physicians or providers are assured a greater supply of patients. PPOs do not replace conventional insurance and may be in competition with HMOs. The providers are paid on a prenegotiated basis, and some are even owners of or investors in the organization. Choice of practitioners may be greater, although the financial incentives of lower deductibles or copayments tend to assure the patient's use of PPO physicians.

Fee-for-service is the traditional form of payment for providing medical care. An individual physician charges for specific procedures or care rendered to an individual patient. It is criticized as lacking comprehensive care or supervision of quality of care. Also, it does not provide cost-containment measures and efficiencies and basically charges whatever the "traffic will bear."

481–483. The answers are 481-C, 482-C, 483-D. *(Rosen, pp 390–399.)* Social Security disability awards are highest for mental and musculoskeletal disorders with back pain disabilities increasing at a rate more than ten times the growth of our population. The greatest number of Social Security disability awards for women are for mental disorders. The greatest number of awards for men and women combined are also for mental disorders. Of the various kinds of disability, back pain and mental disorders are most affected by the external contingencies of eligibility for wage replacement funding (WRF), duration of benefits, and percentage of WRF. These contingencies all influence the persistence of disability.

484–486. The answers are 484-B, 485-C, 486-A. *(U.S. Public Health Service, pp 1–8.)* Heart disease is still the leading cause of death in the U.S. It reached a peak before 1950, but has continued to decline since then. Between 1980 and 1991 the death rate for heart disease decreased by 27 percent (from 202 to 148.2 deaths per 100,000 population).

Malignant neoplasms increased about 1 percent between 1980 and 1991, from 132.8 per 100,000 population in 1980 to 134.5 in 1991. Lung cancer increased 10 percent for white males and 5 percent for black males. In 1988 the incidence of lung cancer in women exceeded the incidence of breast cancer (formerly the highest form of cancer in women), and lung cancer is expected to continue to increase over the next decade because of the increased smoking behavior of women.

Mortality from chronic obstructive pulmonary disease has increased by 26 percent (from 15.9 to 20.1 deaths per 100,000 population). This has primarily resulted from smoking behaviors. It has now become the fourth leading cause of death in the U.S., and it is increasing most rapidly in women (a 45 percent increase in men versus a 79 percent increase in women).

Mortality from cerebrovascular diseases declined by 34 percent between 1980 and 1991. It is still the third leading cause of death in the U.S. The present rate is 26.8 deaths per 100,000 population down from 40.8. The annual rate of decrease has been about 5 percent per year since 1970 for both sexes and major race groups. Better control of hypertension and healthier cardiovascular systems are given as explanations. However, the death rate for black males and females is almost twice that for white males and females.

The suicide rate has held rather constant with 11.4 deaths per 100,000 population in 1980 and 11.4 in 1991, although it has varied within subgroups such as adolescents and the elderly. It is the second leading cause (after accidents) of death among those 15 to 24 years of age. The youth suicide rate more than tripled between 1950 and 1991. White males committed the majority of suicides in all age groups. The male-to-female ratio was 5 to 1, and the white-to-black ratio was almost 2 to 1. Homicide is the second leading cause of death for black children, with a death rate 3 to 4 times the rate for any other group. The homicide rate for black adolescents continues to rise.

Behavioral Statistics and Design

DIRECTIONS: Each question below contains five suggested responses. Select the **one best** response to each question.

487. In studying human development, the remeasurement of a cross-sectional sample of people after a given fixed interval of time has passed is called

(A) time-lag design
(B) sequential design
(C) multivariate design
(D) cross-sectional design
(E) longitudinal design

488. If one is conducting research that requires comparisons of content and material gathered for certain patients by different interviewers, the best format to use would be one that is

(A) projective
(B) structured
(C) unstructured
(D) analytical
(E) none of the above

489. The revised third edition and subsequent fourth edition of the *Diagnostic and Statistical Manual of Mental Disorders (DSM)* offer an improvement over earlier psychiatric classifications. Their major advantage is that they

(A) identify mental illness as a disease
(B) deal with predisposing factors
(C) confirm and support the nosologic system
(D) present an all-inclusive classification system
(E) present a multiaxial classification system

490. Which of the following statements best describes the Likert technique of attitude measurement?

(A) Subjects indicate on five-point scales the extent of their agreement with a set of attitude statements

(B) Subjects indicate whether they agree with each of a series of attitude statements, which are equally spaced along an attitude continuum

(C) Subjects' responses to an open-ended interview are coded by content analysis

(D) Subjects judge a particular concept on a series of bipolar semantic scales

(E) Subjects check all acceptable items in a set of statements arranged in order of "difficulty of acceptance"

491. A sample of a population selected so that each observation or unit has an equal chance of being included is called a

(A) random population parameter
(B) systematic sample
(C) systematic random sample
(D) selected sample
(E) simple random sample

492. In research involving follow-up of patients in treatment, the greatest bias in the results is from

(A) sampling error
(B) attrition
(C) incomplete questionnaire
(D) lack of internal validity responses
(E) lack of compliance

493. A statistical method for comparing categorical kinds of data is the

(A) t-test
(B) standard deviation
(C) analysis of variance
(D) correlation coefficient
(E) chi-square test

494. If in attempting to compare two treatment groups, your analysis rejects the null hypothesis, this means that

(A) there is no difference between the two groups
(B) there is a difference between the two groups
(C) any differences between the two groups that do exist are not valid
(D) your analysis does not have enough power to test your research hypothesis
(E) your research hypothesis is rejected

495. All the following topics are characteristic material for descriptive study EXCEPT

(A) treatment of 50 snakebite victims
(B) cluster of cases of Kaposi's sarcoma
(C) prevalence of HIV in homeless men
(D) comparison of two antianxiety drugs
(E) behavioral science for medical students

496. In a meta-analysis, the included studies should have all the following EXCEPT

(A) uniform diagnostic criteria
(B) similar reliability checks
(C) uniform clinical severity
(D) similar therapy
(E) similar measures of outcome

DIRECTIONS: The group of questions below consists of lettered headings followed by a set of numbered items. For each numbered item select the **one** lettered heading with which it is **most** closely associated. Each lettered heading may be used **once, more than once, or not at all.**

Questions 497–500

For each description below, choose the correct term.

(A) F distribution
(B) Power of a test
(C) Correlation coefficient
(D) Meta-analysis
(E) Validity
(F) Reliability
(G) Standard deviation

497. All values begin at zero and range upward to positive infinity

498. A measure of the degree or strength of association between two variables

499. The degree to which an instrument measures what it is supposed to measure

500. The degree to which results are consistent on a repeat measurement

Behavioral Statistics
and Design
Answers

487. The answer is B. *(Lerner, Psychology, pp 171–179.)* The four research designs for studying human growth and development are longitudinal, cross-sectional, time-lag, and sequential. In the longitudinal design, the same group of people are observed at more than one time. The cross-sectional design studies age groups at one time. The time-lag design allows a researcher to see differences in behavior associated with particular ages at various times in history. Instead of focusing on one cohort or one time of measurement, a time-lag design considers only one age level at different times of measurement, say 1950, 1960, 1970, and 1980. The sequential design combines features of longitudinal and cross-sectional designs so that the researcher may assess differences between groups owing to age, cohort, or time of testing. The sequential design involves the remeasurement of a cross-sectional sample of people after a given fixed interval of time, obtaining repeated measures from each of the different cohort groups included in a given cross-sectional sample, and obtaining data from retest control groups to assess the effects of retesting.

488. The answer is B. *(Gatchel, 2/e, pp 200–203.)* The clinical interview is effective in obtaining data on concerns, feelings, problems, and history, but it tends to vary depending on the clinical and theoretical orientation of the interviewer, e.g., behavioral versus psychoanalytical. If one must compare the data gathered by different interviewers, interviewer bias can be reduced by using a rather highly structured interview of predetermined questions with specific categories of analysis or by using an existing standardized test, questionnaire, or rating scale. An audiotaped analysis could be designed so that a quantitative analysis would allow comparisons using different interviewers, but if the interviews were unstructured, comparisons of content would not be valid. Projective techniques are unstructured because they allow the subject to "project" his or her feelings, attitudes, or interpretations of an ambiguous stimulus or situation. Comparisons of different interviewers would not be valid.

489. The answer is E. *(Gatchel, 2/e, pp 197–200.)* *DSM* presents the official classification schema of mental disorders. Serious problems of validity and reliability were associated with the first two editions of *DSM*. The major advantage that began with the revised third edition was that it allowed for a multiaxial classification. Earlier classifications were one-category systems, with the patient receiving only one diagnostic label or category. *DSM-IV* now provides the possibility that a patient with several disorders can be scored or classified with multiaxial diagnoses. The broad dimensions or axes are as follows: I. Clinical psychiatric syndromes and other conditions; II. Personality disorders (adults) and specific developmental disorders (children and adolescents); III. Physical disorders; IV. Severity of psychosocial stressors; and V. Highest level of adaptive function during the past year.

490. The answer is A. *(Vander Zanden, 4/e, pp 176–177.)* In the Likert "method of summated ratings" relating to attitude measurement, subjects indicate on five-point scales the extent of their agreement with a series of attitude statements. These ratings are then summated to yield a single attitude score. This technique is less laborious than the Thurstone technique (choice B of the question), in which statements are first sorted by a group of judges into 11 equally spaced categories. The Guttman scalogram (choice E) differs from both of these techniques in that it involves a series of items assumed to be cumulative—that is, acceptance of one statement is assumed to imply acceptance of all other less extreme statements. Whereas Guttman assumes unidimensional concepts, C. E. Osgood argues for multidimensionality. His "semantic differential" (choice D) uses a series of seven-point bipolar scales (e.g., good-bad, strong-weak, active-passive) that are answered with respect to a single word or concept.

491. The answer is E. *(Rosenthal, 2/e, pp 205–229.)* When a mean and a standard deviation are calculated by using the data from the entire population, they are called *population parameters*. When they are calculated from a sample of that population they are referred to as *sample statistics*. In choosing a sample, the objective is to select observations or units that are truly representative of the total population being studied. If the sample is selected so that each observation or unit has an equal chance of being included in the sample, it is called a *simple random sample*. Randomness does not mean haphazardness, selecting something without intentional bias, having someone else choose, or using some general techniques, such as "randomly" pointing one's finger or dart throwing. Using a table of random numbers or some mechanical means is considered best. An example of using a systematic sample would be interviewing every third person. Every possible source of sample bias must be explored and eliminated.

492. The answer is B. *(Gehlbach, 3/e, pp 70–73, 104–106.)* The biggest single problem of follow-up design studies is loss through attrition, representing the loss of valuable data and information. Most studies try to prevent sampling bias at the beginning of the study, although it is a frequent bias in medical research, especially when psychosocial factors are ignored. There are many reasons for loss to follow-up (e.g., patients change addresses or fail to respond to questionnaires or phone calls), but it is such a significant source of bias (and disappointment) that follow-up methods should be developed as a part of the original design. Regretably, many AIDS studies suffer from such loss to follow-up bias. Incomplete questionnaires and lack of compliance result in bias, but they can be controlled by planning for adequate follow-up and supervision. Internal validity is confirmed early in a study design when it is determined that results appear to be accurate and the methods and analysis bear-up under scrutiny.

493. The answer is E. *(Gehlbach, 3/e, pp 161–176.)* The chi-square test is used to compare categorical kinds of data (number of patients, two effects, two other measurements) that can be categorized in a 2×2 table, such as comparing two different drugs with high and low fatigue. It will tell whether the two distributions are different enough to indicate that they are not likely to have been drawn from the same population. In other words, the chi-square test tells us whether the differences we observe are real or are an artifact of sampling variability. The *t*-test compares the reliability of the difference between two means (averages) to determine whether the difference could have occurred by chance. A standard deviation shows how much variability there is within a distribution. Analysis of variance is a more complex form of the *t*-test, allowing comparisons among the means of three or more groups. The correlation coefficient evaluates the strengths of linear relationships or association between two variables, e.g., whether patients' weights and blood pressures are related to each other.

494. The answer is B. *(Gehlbach, 3/e, pp 148–149.)* The null hypothesis states that there is no difference between the items (e.g., groups, therapies, drugs, or measurements) being compared. It is used to help you decide whether the differences are real or perhaps just due to the quirks of your sampling. In using the null hypothesis, you are assuming (for statistical purposes) that there is no difference between the two groups or treatments. This is quite different, in fact contrary, to your research hypothesis, which usually states that there is indeed a difference and you are going to prove it. Thus, statistical rejection of the null hypothesis means that your research hypothesis is supported. The 5 percent probability standard is the usual confidence level; it indicates that only a 5 percent probability exists that the difference you found between two groups occurred by chance.

495. The answer is D. *(Gehlbach, 3/e, pp 15–18.)* A descriptive study records events, observations, and activities. It does not provide explanations of causes or present evidence needed to compare and evaluate efficacy of two treatments, drugs, or procedures. The comparison of two antianxiety drugs would be an experimental study, even though it might contain many elements of a descriptive study. Descriptive studies document and communicate experience, ideas, programs, treatments, and observations, but would not provide the data controls and comparisons that would be included in an experimental study. Thus, the treatment of snakebites, cluster of cases, prevalence of HIV, and a course for medical students would be primarily descriptions, not experimental trials, comparisons, or data analyses.

496. The answer is E. *(Gehlbach, 3/e, pp 246–248.)* Meta-analysis is a method of pooling data from several studies to help answer questions that were beyond the power of each study alone. In effect, it increases the sample size, providing more precise estimates of risks or rates; in the case of clinical trials, it also means less likelihood of a type II error. Uniform diagnostic criteria and uniform clinical severity are required to assure that all the patients had the same disease and that the disease was of similar severity. The treatment regimens must also be similar (e.g., the same antibiotic or behavioral therapy), and there must be similar measures of outcome (e.g., negative bacteria cultures or less depression or the same degree of weight loss). Reliability of the measurements (similarity between repeated measurements with the same test) are important, but not a major problem since reliability is included and monitored in the other criteria (e.g., uniform diagnostic criteria or measures of outcome).

497–500. The answers are 497-A, 498-C, 499-E, 500-F. *(Rosenthal, pp 46–48, 60–61, 140–141, 276–278, 324–326, 439–440.)* In *F* distributions all values begin at zero and range upward to positive infinity. Statistical tests that employ the *F* distribution as the theoretical model are called *parametric tests* because they compare parameters estimated from sample distributions rather than the distributions themselves. Consequently, most of the assumptions concerning their use—normally distributed populations, continuous variables, and equal population variances—act to preserve the accuracy of the estimated procedures. There is the additional restriction that the observations must be independent because the computed *F* test value is a ratio of explained to unexplained variance. Any correlation between the observations would make such a ratio meaningless.

Power is the probability of rejecting the null hypothesis when the null hypothesis is false. Your hope, according to your hypothesis, is that you will be able to reject the null hypothesis. The sample size can be increased if the preliminary calculations indicate that the power is inadequate. Power can also be increased by reconstructing the experimental design to provide a more precise estimate of the treatment effects and smaller error effects.

A correlation analysis is used to obtain a measure of the degree or strength of association between two variables under study. The degree of association between X and Y is provided by r, the coefficient of correlation. It is important to observe several precautions: (1) the relationship between variables must be linear, (2) there is a real danger of making inferences beyond the range of actual observations or measurements on which the analysis is based, and (3) it must always be remembered that correlation does not necessarily mean causation. A significant correlation is an indication that the two variables, X and Y, tend to be associated. The problem is that a third variable may be affecting the relationship, thus causing both X and Y to vary together.

A meta-analysis is the quantitative analysis of the results of a group of studies of a given topic, i.e., an analysis of analyses. It is a widely used set of statistical procedures for comparing and combining results from different studies. One of the advantages of meta-analysis is that by combining the results of a number of studies we can increase the power of the statistical analysis, thus allowing us to identify effects that might escape our notice in a single study.

Reliability is the degree to which the results of one measurement are consistent (stable) upon repetition of the measurement or experiment. The term *reliability coefficient* refers to the degree to which what you have measured is relatively free of measurement fluctuations. Reliability coefficient would tell us about the objectivity or repeatability of our observations, judgments, or ratings.

Validity tells us the degree to which a test or questionnaire is measuring what it is supposed to be measuring. It is the most important consideration in test evaluation. We would have to have evidence in four categories: (1) content-related validity (e.g., Does the test contain items from the appropriate content areas?); (2) criterion validity, or the degree to which the test correlates with the outcome criteria (e.g., those things a medical student should know); (3) concurrent validity, which is a correlation of the results of the test with the concurrent performance or task being assessed; and (4) predictive validity, a correlation of the extent to which the test predicts the outcome or future performance (e.g., graduation).

Bibliography

Ader R, Felton DL, Cohen N (eds): *Psychoneuroimmunology,* 2/e. New York, Academic Press, 1991

Carlson NR: *Physiology of Behavior,* 4/e. Boston, Allyn & Bacon, 1991.

Conger JJ: *Adolescence and Youth: Psychological Development in a Changing World,* 4/e. New York, Harper & Row, 1991.

Feuerstein M, Labbe EE, Kuczmierczyk AR: *Health Psychology: A Psychobiological Perspective.* New York, Plenum, 1986.

Gatchel RJ, Baum A, Krantz DS: *An Introduction to Health Psychology,* 2/e. New York, Random House, 1989.

Gehlbach SH: *Interpreting the Medical Literature,* 3/e. New York, McGraw-Hill, 1993.

Hamburg DA, Sartorius N: *Health and Behavior: Selected Perspectives.* New York, Cambridge University, 1989.

Hazzard WR, et al: *Principles of Geriatric Medicine and Gerontology,* 3/e. New York, McGraw-Hill, 1994.

Isselbacher KJ, et al (eds): *Harrison's Principles of Internal Medicine,* 13/e. New York, McGraw-Hill, 1994.

Kandel ER, Schwartz JH (eds): *Principles of Neural Science,* 3/e. New York, Elsevier, 1991.

Kaplan HL, Sadock BJ, Grebb JA: *Synopsis of Psychiatry,* 7/e. Baltimore, Williams & Wilkins, 1994.

Kaptein AA, et al (eds): *Behavioral Medicine: Psychological Treatment of Somatic Disorders.* New York, John Wiley & Sons, 1990.

Last JM (ed): *Maxcy-Rosenau Public Health and Preventive Medicine,* 13/e. East Norwalk, CT, Appleton & Lange, 1992.

Lerner RM, et al (eds): *Encyclopedia of Adolescence.* New York, Garland, 1991.

Lerner RM, et al: *Psychology.* New York, Macmillan, 1986.

Linden W (ed): *Biological Barriers in Behavioral Medicine.* New York, Plenum, 1988.

Lindzey G, Aronson A (eds): *The Handbook of Social Psychology,* vol 2, 3/e, New York, Random House, 1985.

Plomin R, DeFries JJ, McClearn GE: *Behavioral Genetics: A Primer,* 2/e. San Francisco, WH Freeman, 1990.

Rosen JC, Soloman LJ (eds): *Prevention in Health Psychology.* Hanover, NH, University Press of New England, 1985.

Rosenthal R, Rosnow R: *Essentials of Behavioral Research: Methods and Data Analysis,* 2/e. New York, McGraw-Hill, 1991.

Schneiderman N, Tapp J: *Behavioral Medicine: The Bio-Psychosocial Approach.* Hillsdale, NJ, Lawrence Erlbaum, 1985.

Schuster CS, Ashburn SS: *The Process of Human Development: A Holistic Approach,* 3/e. Boston, Little, Brown, 1992.

Sierles FS (ed): *Behavioral Science for Medical Students,* Baltimore, Williams & Wilkins, 1993.

Simons RD (ed): *Understanding Human Behavior in Health and Illness,* 3/e. Baltimore, Williams & Wilkins, 1985.

Twaddle AC, Hessler RM: *A Sociology of Health,* 2/e. New York, Macmillan, 1986.

U.S. Public Health Service: *Health United States, 1994,* PHS No. 94–1232. Washington, D.C., U.S. Department of Health and Human Services, 1994.

Vander Zanden JW: *Social Psychology,* 4/e. New York, Random House, 1987.

Williams RB: *Perspectives on Behavioral Medicine: Neuroendocrine Control and Behavior,* vol 2. New York, Academic Press, 1985.

Williams SJ, Torrens PR: *Introduction to Health Services,* 3/e. New York, John Wiley & Sons, 1989.